MRCP PART 1 PAEDIATRIC PAST TOPICS

A REVISION SYLLABUS AND MCQ PRACTICE EXAM

Compiled and edited by

David Goldblatt MRCP PhD
Senior Lecturer/Honorary Consultant
Institute of Child Health
and Great Ormond Street Hospital
for Children NHS Trust
University College London Medical School

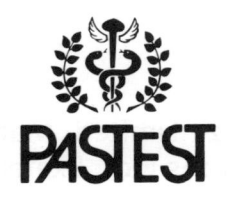

PASTEST

© PasTest 1997
Egerton Court, Parkgate Estate, Knutsford, Cheshire
WA16 8DX

All rights reserved. No part of this publication may be reproduced, stored in a retrieval system, or transmitted, in any form or by any means, electronic, mechanical, photocopying, recording or otherwise without the prior permission of the copyright owner.

First published 1997

ISBN 1 901198 00 6

A catalogue record for this book is available from the British Library.

Text prepared by Breeze Limited, Manchester.
Printed by BPC Wheatons Ltd., Exeter

CONTENTS

Foreword	v
Basic Science	1
Cardiology	6
Dermatology	11
Ear, Nose and Throat	11
Embryology	12
Endocrinology	14
Gastroenterology	16
General Paediatrics	19
Genetics	20
Growth and Development	23
Haematology and Oncology	27
Immunology	32
Infectious Diseases	35
Metabolic Disease	42
Neonatology	45
Nephrology	49
Neurology	52
Nutrition	58
Ophthalmology	59
Pharmacology	60
Psychiatry	64
Respiratory Disease	68
Rheumatology	72
Statistics	73
MCQ Practice Examination	74
Answers to Practice Examination	90
PasTest Revision Books for MRCP Part 1 Paediatrics	105
PasTest Courses for MRCP Part 1 Paediatrics	106

THE PAEDIATRIC MRCP PART 1 EXAMINATION

A breakdown of the relative distribution of topics is given below. A slight variation may occur from exam to exam.

Subject Area	Number of MCQs
Neurology	5
Infectious Diseases	5
Cardiology	5
Respiratory	4
Haematology/Oncology	4
Growth/Development	3
Psychiatry/Sexual Abuse	3
Neonatology	3
Gastroenterology	3
Endocrinology	3
Immunology	3
Nephrology	3
Pharmacology	2
General Paediatrics	2
Inborn Errors	2
Genetics	2
Embryology/Fetal Medicine	1
Nutrition	1
Ophthalmology	1
Rheumatology	1
Statistics	1
Surgery	1
ENT	1
Mediators	1
Total Number of MCQs	**60**

FOREWORD

Higher training in paediatrics requires completion of Part 1 and Part 2 of the paediatric Membership exams. The Paediatric MRCP Part 1 was introduced in October 1993 as an exam consisting of 30 paediatric questions and 30 questions which were common to both paediatrics and general medicine. Since its introduction, the exam has become progressively more paediatric in its orientation and paediatricians are no longer at a disadvantage. An intensive training course was developed by PasTest for the first paediatric exam and has continued three times a year ever since. The exam content is continually analysed by PasTest and the course lecturers, and is reflected in the core material, lectures and practice exams used on the course. This experience has also been utilised in the production of PasTest's paediatric MCQ books and in this book, a revision syllabus for paediatric MRCP Part 1.

It is unwise to be too prescriptive about the optimum preparation for passing this exam as candidates differ in their knowledge base and ability to perform in MCQ exams. However, to pass this exam candidates should ideally (1) allow adequate time to revise and prepare for the exam, (2) attend a revision course, (3) practice typical MCQs and (4) be familiar with the range of topics usually tested. This book contains data carefully compiled by Dr Goldblatt on the content and topics frequently found in the exam. The material has been accumulated by amalgamating the feedback from candidates who have taken the exam after attending PasTest courses from October 1993 to September 1996. It is an invaluable resource, providing all prospective Membership candidates with the information required to organise an effective revision timetable.

Foreword

How to use this book

The material is displayed in three ways:

Topics are listed chronologically within each subject area. For each subject, specific topics are listed in order of frequency. Finally a checklist has been compiled for each subject under more general headings to aid revision planning.

This format enables candidates to efficiently analyse the range of topics tested, highlighting the changes in examination content over the last three years. The frequency index and checklists help candidates to effectively direct their limited revision time towards more popular topics. Finally, having revised the topics set out in this book, candidates should test their ability by sitting the typical exam which can be found towards the end of this book. It is recommended that this should be performed under simulated examination conditions, referring to the detailed answers only when the exam time is up.

We would like to thank all PasTest course attenders for their invaluable feedback, without which this book would not have been possible.

Dr Nigel Klein
Senior Lecturer and Consultant in Immunology and Infectious Diseases
Great Ormond Street Hospital for Children NHS Trust

BASIC SCIENCE: EXAM TOPICS

July 1996
    Nitric oxide
    Mechanism of Vitamin D

February 1996
    Gastric acid control

October 1995
    Gut hormones
    Vitamin K
    Receptor defects
    Tumour necrosis factor

July 1995
    Steroid hormone receptors
    H_2 receptors
    Atrial natriuretic peptide

February 1995
    Amiodarone
    Cholera toxin
    $Alpha_1$-antitrypsin
    Vitamin D

October 1994
    Mediators of the febrile response
    Polymerase chain reaction
    Insulin
    Nitric oxide
    Mitochondrial DNA

Basic Science

July 1994
- Thyroid hormone
- Vitamin D
- Chloride depletion
- Urine concentration
- Leukotrienes
- Transfer factor
- Iron metabolism

February 1994
- Somatostatin
- Renal physiology
- Gut absorption of micronutrients

October 1993
- Atrial natriuretic peptide
- Oxygen uptake

BASIC SCIENCE: TOPIC FREQUENCY INDEX

Vitamin D	July 1996, Feb 1995, July 1994
Atrial natriuretic peptide	July 1995, Oct 1995
Nitric oxide	July 1996, Oct 1994
Alpha$_1$-antitrypsin	Feb 1995
Amiodarone	Feb 1995
Chloride depletion	July 1994
Cholera toxin	Feb 1995
Gastric acid control	Feb 1996
Gut absorbtion of micronutrients	Feb 1994
Gut hormones	Oct 1995
H$_2$ receptors	July 1995
Insulin	Oct 1994
Iron metabolism	July 1994
Leukotrienes	July 1994
Mediators of the febrile response	Oct 1994
Mitochondrial DNA	Oct 1994
Oxygen uptake	Oct 1993
Polymerase chain reaction	Oct 1994
Receptor defects	Oct 1995
Renal physiology	Feb 1994
Somatostatin	Feb 1994
Steroid hormone receptors	July 1995
Thyroid hormone	July 1994
Transfer factor	July 1994
Tumour necrosis factor	Oct 1995
Urine concentration	July 1994
Vitamin K	Oct 1995

BASIC SCIENCE: REVISION CHECKLIST

A fundamental understanding of the scientific basis of diseases is increasingly being expected of candidates. This is reflected in the appearance of questions where at least one of the five options for any given stem will draw on the candidate's understanding of the basic mechanisms of the disease in question. On average 3–4 questions per exam will expect an understanding of basic mechanisms of disease. Numbers in brackets indicate the relative frequency of topics.

Hormones and mediators
- [ ] Atrial natriuretic peptide (2)
- [ ] Nitric oxide (2)
- [ ] Alpha$_1$-antitrypsin
- [ ] Amiodarone
- [ ] Gut hormones
- [ ] H$_2$ receptors
- [ ] Insulin
- [ ] Somatostatin
- [ ] Steroid hormone receptors
- [ ] Thyroid hormone

Immunological mediators
- [ ] Mediators of the febrile response
- [ ] Leukotrienes
- [ ] Tumour necrosis factor
- [ ] Cholera toxin

Vitamins
- [ ] Vitamin D (3)
- [ ] Vitamin K

Basic Science

Physiology
- ☐ Transfer factor
- ☐ Renal physiology
- ☐ Oxygen uptake
- ☐ Iron metabolism
- ☐ Urine concentration
- ☐ Chloride depletion
- ☐ Gastric acid control
- ☐ Gut absorption of micronutrients
- ☐ Receptor defects

Molecular biology
- ☐ Polymerase chain reaction
- ☐ Mitochondrial DNA

CARDIOLOGY: EXAM TOPICS

July 1996
    Fainting after exercise
    Wolff-Parkinson-White syndrome
    Neonatal congestive cardiac failure
    Ostium secundum ASD

February 1996
    Murmur in a 5-year-old
    Cannon 'a' waves
    Neonatal cyanotic heart disease

October 1995
    Wolff-Parkinson-White syndrome
    Heart failure in infancy
    Associations with increased pulmonary flow
    Cyanotic heart disease
    Plethoric lung fields

July 1995
    Wolff-Parkinson-White syndrome
    Ostium secundum ASD
    Patent ductus arteriosus

February 1995
    Fallot's tetralogy
    Heart failure in infancy
    Abnormal vascular rings
    Conditions associated with structural heart defects

October 1994
    Heart sounds
    Cyanotic heart disease
    Ventricular tachycardia

Cardiology

July 1994
- Ductus arteriosus
- Jugular venous pressure

February 1994
- Treatment of supraventricular tachycardia
- Innocent heart murmurs
- Right to left shunts
- Cardiac tamponade
- Coarctation of the aorta

October 1993
- Heart sounds
- Pulmonary artery pressure
- Constrictive pericarditis
- Mitral valve prolapse

CARDIOLOGY: TOPIC FREQUENCY INDEX

Wolff-Parkinson-White	July 1996, Oct 1995, July 1995
Cyanotic heart disease	Oct 1995, Oct 1994 x2
Heart failure in infancy	Oct 1995, Feb 1995
Heart sounds	Oct 1994, Oct 1993
Innocent heart murmurs	Feb 1996, Feb 1994
Jugular venous pressure	Feb 1996, July 1994
Ostium secundum ASD	July 1996, July 1995
Abnormal vascular rings	Feb 1995
Associations with increased pulmonary flow	Oct 1995
Cardiac tamponade	Feb 1994
Coarctation of the aorta	Feb 1994
Conditions associated with structural heart defects	Feb 1995
Constrictive pericarditis	Oct 1993
Ductus arteriosus	July 1994
Fainting after exercise	July 1996
Fallot's tetralogy	Feb 1995
Mitral valve prolapse	Oct 1993
Neonatal congestive cardiac failure	July 1996
Neonatal cyanotic heart disease	Feb 1996
Patent ductus arteriosus	July 1995
Plethoric lung fields	Oct 1995
Pulmonary artery pressure	Oct 1993
Right to left shunts	Feb 1994
Treatment of supraventricular tachycardia	Feb 1994
Ventricular tachycardia	Oct 1994

CARDIOLOGY: REVISION CHECKLIST

Average of five questions per exam. Numbers in brackets indicate the relative frequency of topics.

Congenital abnormalities
- [ ] Cyanotic heart disease (3)
- [ ] Ostium secundum ASD (2)
- [ ] Abnormal vascular rings
- [ ] Coarctation of the aorta
- [ ] Conditions associated with structural heart defects
- [ ] Ductus arteriosus
- [ ] Fallot's tetralogy
- [ ] Neonatal cyanotic heart disease
- [ ] Patent ductus arteriosus
- [ ] Right to left shunts

Auscultation and clinical findings
- [ ] Heart failure in infancy (2)
- [ ] Heart sounds (2)
- [ ] Innocent heart murmurs (2)
- [ ] Neonatal congestive cardiac failure
- [ ] Plethoric lung fields

Physiology
- [ ] Jugular venous pressure (2)
- [ ] Associations with increased pulmonary flow
- [ ] Fainting after exercise
- [ ] Pulmonary artery pressure

Arrhythmia
- [ ] Wolff-Parkinson-White syndrome (3)
- [ ] Treatment of supraventricular tachycardia
- [ ] Ventricular tachycardia

Cardiology

Pericardial disease
- ☐ Constrictive pericarditis
- ☐ Cardiac tamponade

Valvular heart disease
- ☐ Mitral valve prolapse

DERMATOLOGY: EXAM TOPICS

Dermatology questions are relatively rare in the examination but the following four conditions have appeared in previous exams.

July 1996
 Erythema multiforme
 Psoriasis

October 1995
 Systemic mastocytosis

October 1994
 Photosensitivity

EAR, NOSE AND THROAT: EXAM TOPICS

ENT questions appear fairly regularly and the major topics that appear are related to hearing, otis media in all its forms and structural abnormalities of the ears, nose and throat.

July 1996
 Glue ear

February 1996
 Tongue abnormalities
 Serous otitis media

July 1995
 Cleft lip and palate

February 1995
 Causes of deafness

October 1994
 Deafness

July 1994
 Infant hearing

EMBRYOLOGY: EXAM TOPICS

July 1996
 Teratogens

February 1996
 Circulation
 Polyhydramnios

October 1995
 Fetal abnormalities
 General embryology

July 1995
 Endoderm derived tissue
 Impaired fetal lung development

February 1995
 Branchial arch maldevelopment

October 1994
 Fetal circulation
 Maternal conditions affecting the newborn
 Fetal lung development

July 1994
 Fetal development

October 1993
 Fetal development

EMBRYOLOGY: TOPIC FREQUENCY INDEX

Fetal development	July 1994, Oct 1993
Branchial arch maldevelopment	Feb 1995
Circulation	Feb 1996
Endoderm derived tissue	July 1995
Fetal abnormalities	Oct 1995
Fetal circulation	Oct 1994
Fetal lung development	Oct 1994
General embryology	Oct 1995
Impaired fetal lung development	July 1995
Maternal conditions affecting the newborn	Oct 1994
Polyhydramnios	Feb 1996
Teratogens	July 1996

EMBRYOLOGY: REVISION CHECKLIST

Average of one question per exam.

Heart and lung development
- [ ] Fetal circulation
- [ ] Fetal lung development
- [ ] Circulation
- [ ] Impaired fetal lung development

General
- [ ] Origin of fetal tissues
- [ ] Branchial arch maldevelopment
- [ ] Endoderm derived tissue

Maternal-fetal interactions
- [ ] Maternal conditions affecting the newborn
- [ ] Polyhdramnios
- [ ] Teratogens

ENDOCRINOLOGY: EXAM TOPICS

July 1996
Anorexia nervosa

February 1996
Anorexia nervosa
Calcitonin
Diabetes mellitus in a 10-year-old

October 1995
Insulin dependent diabetes mellitus
Short stature

July 1995
Raised PTH levels
Childhood diabetes

February 1995
Insulin dependent diabetes mellitus

October 1994
Delayed bone age

July 1994
Insulin dependent diabetes mellitus

February 1994
Anorexia nervosa
Diabetic ketoacidosis

October 1993
Insulin dependent diabetes mellitus
Pituitary hormones
Polycystic ovarian syndrome

ENDOCRINOLOGY: TOPIC FREQUENCY INDEX

Insulin dependent   Feb 1996, Oct 1995,
  diabetes mellitus   July 1995, Feb 1995,
                             July 1994, Oct 1993
Anorexia nervosa   July 1996, Feb 1996,
                             Feb 1994
Calcitonin   Feb 1996
Delayed bone age   Oct 1994
Diabetes mellitus in a 10-year-old Feb 1996
Diabetic ketoacidosis   Feb 1994
Pituitary hormones   Oct 1993
Polycystic ovarian syndrome Oct 1993
Raised PTH levels   July 1995
Short stature   Oct 1995

ENDOCRINOLOGY: REVISION CHECKLIST

Average of three questions per exam. Questions of an endocrine nature may also be found in other specialties such as gastroenterology. Numbers in brackets indicate the relative frequency of topics.

Diabetes
☐ Insulin dependent diabetes mellitus (7)

Bone and calcium metabolism
☐ Calcitonin
☐ Delayed bone age
☐ Raised PTH levels
☐ Short stature

Miscellaneous
☐ Anorexia nervosa (3)
☐ Pituitary hormones
☐ Polycystic ovarian syndrome

GASTROENTEROLOGY: EXAM TOPICS

July 1996
    Conjugated hyperbilirubinaemia
    Non-infectious diarrhoea in a 3-month-old
    Bile stained vomiting

February 1996
    Unconjugated hyperbilirubinaemia
    Ulcerative colitis
    Projectile vomiting
    Bloody diarrhoea in childhood
    Abdominal pain

October 1995
    Non-bloody diarrhoea

July 1995
    Bloody diarrhoea in childhood
    Unconjugated hyperbilirubinaemia

February 1995
    Crohn's disease
    Flattened small bowel mucosa

October 1994
    Vomiting in a 3-week-old child
    Necrotising enterocolitis
    Gluten enteropathy

July 1994
    Intussusception
    Ulcerative colitis
    Acute pancreatitis

Gastroenterology

February 1994
   Coeliac disease
   Helicobacter pylori

October 1993
   Bloody diarrhoea in childhood
   Crohn's disease

GASTROENTEROLOGY: TOPIC FREQUENCY INDEX

Bloody diarrhoea in childhood	Feb 1996, July 1995, Oct 1993
Coeliac disease	Feb 1995, Oct 1994, Feb 1994
Crohn's disease	Feb 1995, Oct 1993
Unconjugated hyperbilirubinaemia	Feb 1996, July 1995
Abdominal pain	Feb 1996
Acute pancreatitis	July 1994
Bile stained vomiting	July 1996
Conjugated hyperbilirubinaemia	July 1996
Helicobacter pylori	Feb 1994
Intussusception	July 1994
Necrotising enterocolitis	Oct 1994
Non-bloody diarrhoea	Oct 1995
Non-infectious diarrhoea in a 3-month-old	July 1996
Projectile vomiting	Feb 1996
Ulcerative colitis	Feb 1996, July 1994
Vomiting in a 3-week-old child	Oct 1994

GASTROENTEROLOGY: REVISION CHECKLIST

Average of three questions per exam. Numbers in brackets indicate the relative frequency of topics.

Diarrhoea, vomiting and abdominal pain
- [ ] Bloody diarrhoea in childhood (3)
- [ ] Abdominal pain
- [ ] Bile stained vomiting
- [ ] Necrotising enterocolitis
- [ ] Non-bloody diarrhoea
- [ ] Non-infectious diarrhoea in a 3-month-old
- [ ] Projectile vomiting
- [ ] Vomiting in a 3-week-old child

Small/large bowel disease
- [ ] Coeliac disease (3)
- [ ] Crohn's disease (2)
- [ ] Ulcerative colitis

Liver disease
- [ ] Conjugated hyperbilirubinaemia
- [ ] Unconjugated hyperbilirubinaemia (2)

Miscellaneous
- [ ] Acute pancreatitis
- [ ] *Helicobacter pylori*
- [ ] Intussusception

GENERAL PAEDIATRICS: EXAM TOPICS

This category contains questions that do not fit into the other major subspecialties included in the breakdown of the examination. They can best be described as those relevant to general paediatrics or paediatric surgery and one can expect at least one such question per examination.

October 1995
Umbilical hernias

July 1995
Decreased neck mobility
Scrotal swellings

February 1995
Acute appendicitis

October 1994
Splenomegaly

July 1994
Sudden death
Sudden infant death syndrome
Medical contraindications to adoption

February 1994
Congenital dislocation of the hip
Osteolytic lesions in a 2-year-old
Abdominal pain
Intussusception

October 1993
Surgical conditions at 3 months of age
Contraindications to swimming

GENETICS: EXAM TOPICS

July 1996
X-linked recessive inheritance

February 1996
X-linked dominant inheritance
Klinefelter's syndrome

October 1995
Klinefelter's syndrome
Down's syndrome
Autosomal dominant conditions

July 1995
Chromosome defects
Turner's syndrome
Fragile X syndrome
Prader Willi syndrome

February 1995
Genetic anticipation
Autosomal dominant conditions

October 1994
Marfan's syndrome

July 1994
Duchenne muscular dystrophy

February 1994
Autosomal recessive conditions

Genetics

October 1993
  Mental subnormality
  Noonan's syndrome
  Duchenne muscular dystrophy

GENETICS: TOPIC FREQUENCY INDEX

Autosomal dominant conditions	Oct 1995, Feb 1995,
Duchenne muscular dystrophy	July 1994, Oct 1993
Klinefelter's syndrome	Feb 1996, Oct 1995
Autosomal recessive conditions	Feb 1994
Chromosome defects	July 1995
Down's syndrome	Oct 1995
Fragile X	July 1995
Genetic anticipation	Feb 1995
Marfan's syndrome	Oct 1994
Mental subnormality	Oct 1993
Noonan's syndrome	Oct 1993
Prader Willi syndrome	July 1995
Turner's syndrome	July 1995
X-linked dominant inheritance	Feb 1996
X-linked recessive inheritance	July 1996

GENETICS: REVISION CHECKLIST

Average of one question per exam. Every exam contains at least one genetics question. Numbers in brackets indicate the relative frequency of topics.

Syndromes
- [ ] Duchenne muscular dystrophy (2)
- [ ] Klinefelter's syndrome (2)
- [ ] Down's syndrome
- [ ] Fragile X
- [ ] Marfan's syndrome
- [ ] Mental subnormality
- [ ] Noonan's syndrome
- [ ] Prader Willi syndrome
- [ ] Turner's syndrome
- [ ] Chromosome defects

Modes of inheritance
- [ ] Autosomal dominant conditions (2)
- [ ] Autosomal recessive conditions
- [ ] X-linked dominant conditions
- [ ] X-linked recessive conditions

Miscellaneous
- [ ] Genetic anticipation

GROWTH AND DEVELOPMENT: EXAM TOPICS

July 1996
    2-year-old development
    Specific language delay
    Associations with a large head
    Obesity
    Short stature in a 5-year-old

February 1996
    Causes of learning disabilities
    1-year-old developmental milestones
    Large head in a 9-month-old
    Delayed bone age

October 1995
    3-year-old development
    Delayed speech development
    Cerebral palsy at 9 months of age

July 1995
    Developmental screening
    Growth milestones and normal ranges
    Nocturnal enuresis
    Developmental assessment in a 3-year-old

February 1995
    1-year-old developmental assessment
    Reading in a 7-year-old

October 1994
    3-year-old developmental assessment

Growth and Development

July 1994
- Longitudinal growth
- Precocious puberty
- Puberty
- 2-year-old developmental assessment

February 1994
- 18-month-old development assessment
- 2-year-old development
- Risk factors for developmental delay
- 6-month-old development
- Growth milestones and normal ranges

October 1993
- 2-year-old developmental assessment
- Puberty
- Delayed bone age
- 8-month-old development
- Short stature
- Bone metabolism

GROWTH AND DEVELOPMENT: TOPIC FREQUENCY INDEX

Age-appropriate developmental milestones	July 1996, Feb 1996, Oct 1995, July 1995, Feb 1995, Oct 1994, July 1994, Feb 1994 x3, Oct 1993 x2
Associations with a large head	July 1996, Feb 1996
Delayed bone age	Feb 1996, Oct 1993
Growth milestones and normal ranges	July 1995, Feb 1994
Puberty	July 1994, Oct 1993
Short stature	July 1996, Oct 1993
Bone metabolism	Oct 1993
Causes of learning disabilities	Feb 1996
Cerebral palsy at 9 months of age	Oct 1995
Delayed speech development	Oct 1995
Developmental screening	July 1995
Longitudinal growth	July 1994
Nocturnal enuresis	July 1995
Obesity	July 1996
Precocious puberty	July 1994
Reading in a 7-year-old	Feb 1995
Risk factors for developmental delay	Feb 1994
Specific language delay	July 1996

GROWTH AND DEVELOPMENT: REVISION CHECKLIST

Average of three questions per exam. Every exam contains at least one question on the age-appropriate developmental milestones. Numbers in brackets indicate the relative frequency of topics.

Normal and abnormal developmental assessment
- ☐ Age appropriate developmental milestones (12)
- ☐ Delayed speech development
- ☐ Developmental screening
- ☐ Reading in a 7-year-old
- ☐ Causes of learning disabilities
- ☐ Risk factors for developmental delay
- ☐ Specific language delay

Normal and Abnormal Physical Development
- ☐ Growth milestones and normal range (2)
- ☐ Puberty (2)
- ☐ Delayed bone age (2)
- ☐ Short stature (2)
- ☐ Longitudinal growth
- ☐ Precocious puberty
- ☐ Cerebral palsy at 9 months old

Miscellaneous
- ☐ Associations with a large head (2)
- ☐ Bone metabolism
- ☐ Nocturnal enuresis
- ☐ Obesity

HAEMATOLOGY AND ONCOLOGY: EXAM TOPICS

July 1996
   Leukaemia
   Thalassaemia major

February 1996
   Causes of a prolonged bleeding time
   Causes of a raised reticulocyte count
   Iron therapy
   Wilm's tumour

October 1995
   Osteolytic bone lesions
   Body iron stores
   Causes of pancytopenia and splenomegaly
   ABO incompatibility

July 1995
   Von Willebrand's disease
   Vitamin K in newborns
   Uses of fresh frozen plasma
   Abnormal haemoglobin synthesis
   Hyposplenism

February 1995
   Red cell folate
   Chronic intravascular haemolysis
   Acute lymphoblastic leukaemia

October 1994
   Anaemia in a 5-year-old
   Hodgkin's disease
   Leukaemia

July 1994
- Iron toxicity
- Sickle cell disease
- Hereditary spherocytosis

February 1994
- Idiopathic thrombocytopenic purpura
- Haemolytic anaemia
- Sickle cell disease
- Haemoglobinuria

October 1993
- CNS tumours
- Anaemia
- Splenectomy
- Haem biosynthesis

HAEMATOLOGY AND ONCOLOGY: TOPIC FREQUENCY INDEX

Leukaemia	July 1996, Feb 1995, Oct 1994
Anaemia	Oct 1994, Oct 1993
Sickle cell disease	July 1994, Feb 1994
Abnormal haemaglobin synthesis	July 1995
ABO incompatibility	Oct 1995
Body iron stores	Oct 1995
Causes of a prolonged bleeding time	Feb 1996
Causes of a raised reticulocyte count	Feb 1996
Causes of pancytopenia and splenomegaly	Oct 1995
Chronic intravascular haemolysis	Feb 1995
CNS tumours	Oct 1993
Haem biosynthesis	Oct 1993
Haemoglobinuria	Feb 1994
Haemolytic anaemia	Feb 1994
Hereditary spherocytosis	July 1994
Hodgkin's disease	Oct 1994
Hyposplenism	July 1995
Idiopathic thrombocytopenic purpura	Feb 1994
Iron therapy	Feb 1996
Iron toxicity	July 1994
Osteolytic bone lesions	Oct 1995
Red cell folate	Feb 1995
Splenectomy	Oct 1993
Thalassaemia major	July 1996
Uses of fresh frozen plasma	July 1995
Vitamin K in newborns	July 1995
Von Willebrand's disease	July 1995
Wilm's tumour	Feb 1996

HAEMATOLOGY AND ONCOLOGY: REVISION CHECKLIST

Average of four questions per exam. Numbers in brackets indicate the relative frequency of topics.

Haemostasis
- [ ] Causes of a prolonged bleeding time
- [ ] Chronic intravascular haemolysis
- [x] Idiopathic thrombocytopenic purpura
- [ ] Vitamin K in newborns
- [x] Uses of fresh frozen plasma
- [ ] Von Willebrand's disease

Oncology
- [x] Leukaemia (3)
- [ ] CNS tumours
- [x] Hodgkin's disease
- [ ] Wilm's tumour
- [ ] Osteolytic bone lesions

Anaemia
- [x] Anaemia (2)
- [x] Haemolytic anaemia
- [x] Red cell folate

Haemoglobinopathies
- [x] Sickle cell disease (2)
- [ ] Abnormal haemoglobin synthesis
- [x] Hereditary spherocytosis
- [x] Thalassaemia major

Iron and haemoglobin physiology
- [x] Body iron stores
- [ ] Haem biosynthesis
- [ ] Haemoglobinuria
- [x] Iron therapy

Haematology and Oncology

- [x] Iron toxicity

Miscellaneous
- [ ] ABO incompatibility
- [ ] Causes of a raised reticulocyte count
- [ ] Causes of pancytopenia and splenomegaly
- [ ] Hyposplenism
- [ ] Splenectomy

IMMUNOLOGY: EXAM TOPICS

July 1996
>Complement
>Fc portion of IgG

February 1996
>Complement in systemic disease
>Newborn immunity
>T cell deficiency
>Childhood immunisations

October 1995
>Breast milk contents

July 1995
>Gamma-interferon
>Allograft rejection
>IgE
>Hypersensitivity

February 1995
>Monoclonal gammopathy

October 1994
>T lymphocytes

July 1994
>IgA
>Interferon
>Immune complexes

February 1994
>Monoclonal antibodies
>Hereditary angio-oedema

Immunology

October 1993
- Haemophilus vaccines
- Major histocompatibility complex
- Allergic reactions

IMMUNOLOGY: TOPIC FREQUENCY INDEX

Allergic reactions	Oct 1993
Allograft rejection	July 1995
Breast milk contents	Oct 1995
Childhood immunisations	Feb 1996
Complement	July 1996
Complement in systemic disease	Feb 1996
Fc portion of IgG	July 1996
Gamma-interferon	July 1995
Haemophilus vaccines	Oct 1993
Hereditary angio-oedema	Feb 1994
Hypersensitivity	July 1995
IgA	July 1994
IgE	July 1995
Immune complexes	July 1994
Interferon	July 1994
Major histocompatibility complex	Oct 1993
Monoclonal antibodies	Feb 1994
Monoclonal gammopathy	Feb 1995
Newborn immunity	Feb 1996
T cell deficiency	Feb 1996
T lymphocytes	Oct 1994

IMMUNOLOGY: REVISION CHECKLIST

An average of three immunology questions appear in each exam.

Cellular immunity
- [ ] Allograft rejection
- [ ] T cell deficiency
- [ ] T lymphocytes
- [ ] Major histocompatibility complex

Antibodies and complement
- [ ] IgA
- [ ] IgE
- [ ] Immune complexes
- [ ] Fc portion of IgG
- [ ] Complement
- [ ] Complement in systemic disease
- [ ] Hereditary angio-oedema
- [ ] Monoclonal antibodies
- [ ] Monoclonal gammopathy

Cytokines
- [ ] Gamma-interferon
- [ ] Interferon

Allergy and hypersensitivity
- [ ] Allergic reactions
- [ ] Hypersensitivity

Miscellaneous
- [ ] Breast milk contents
- [ ] Childhood immunisations
- [ ] Haemophilus vaccines
- [ ] Newborn immunity

INFECTIOUS DISEASES: EXAM TOPICS

July 1996
- Cholera
- Influenza vaccination
- Acquired toxoplasmosis
- Mumps
- Hepatitis
- Paediatric HIV
- Infectious mononucleosis
- Epiglottitis

February 1996
- HIV transmission
- *Chlamydia trachomatis*
- Rubella
- Adenovirus
- Kawasaki's disease
- Malaria

October 1995
- Congenital toxoplasmosis
- *Mycoplasma pneumoniae*
- Infectious mononucleosis
- Brucellosis
- Toxin-mediated staphylococcal infection

July 1995
- Antibiotic prophylaxis
- Malaria
- Parvovirus B19
- Immunisation
- Tonsillar exudates
- *Erythema infectiosum*

Infectious Diseases

February 1995
- Chicken pox
- Post-splenectomy septicaemia
- Tuberculosis
- Malaria
- Hepatitis C
- HIV

October 1994
- Influenza vaccination
- HIV
- Hepatitis B
- *Pneumocystis carinii*
- Cerebral abscess
- Malaria
- CNS involvement in HIV
- Tetanus

July 1994
- Infectious causes of hydrops fetalis
- Measles
- Infections associated with eosinophilia
- Infectious mononucleosis
- *Giardia lamblia*
- Malaria
- Brucellosis and toxoplasmosis

February 1994
- Pertussis vaccination
- Brucellosis
- Rubella
- Hepatitis C

Infectious Diseases

October 1993
    BCG
    Fever and splenomegaly
    HIV

INFECTIOUS DISEASES: TOPIC FREQUENCY INDEX

HIV	July 1996, Feb 1996, Feb 1995, Oct 1994 x 2, Oct 1993
Malaria	Feb 1996, July 1995, Feb 1995, Oct 1994, July 1994
Brucellosis	Oct 1995, July 1994, Feb 1994
Infectious mononucleosis	July 1996, July 1994, Oct 1995
Acquired toxoplasmosis	July 1996, July 1994
Hepatitis C	Feb 1995, Feb 1994
Influenza vaccination	July 1996, Oct 1994
Rubella	Feb 1996, Feb 1994
Adenovirus	Feb 1996
Antibiotic prophylaxis	July 1995
BCG	Oct 1993
Cerebral abscess	Oct 1994
Chicken pox	Feb 1995
Chlamydia trachomatis	Feb 1996
Cholera	July 1996
Congenital toxoplasmosis	Oct 1995
Epiglottitis	July 1996
Erythema infectiosum	July 1995
Fever and splenomegaly	Oct 1993
Giardia lamblia	July 1994
Hepatitis	July 1996
Hepatitis B	Oct 1994
Immunisation	July 1995
Infections associated with eosinophilia	July 1994
Infectious causes of hydrops fetalis	July 1994
Kawasaki's disease	Feb 1996

Infectious Diseases

Measles	July 1994
Mumps	July 1996
Mycoplasma pneumoniae	Oct 1995
Parvovirus B19	July 1995
Pertussis vaccination	Feb 1994
Pneumocystis carinii	Oct 1994
Post-splenectomy septicaemia	Feb 1995
Tetanus	Oct 1994
Tonsillar exudates	July 1995
Toxin-mediated staphylococcal infection	Oct 1995
Tuberculosis	Feb 1995

INFECTIOUS DISEASES: REVISION CHECKLIST

Infectious diseases is one of the most popular topics and questions cross over with a variety of other sub-specialties such as neurology. An average of five questions appear in each exam. Numbers in brackets indicate the relative frequency of topics.

Viral infections
- [ ] HIV (6)
- [ ] Infectious mononucleosis (3)
- [ ] Hepatitis C (2)
- [ ] Rubella (2)
- [ ] Influenza vaccination (2)
- [ ] Adenovirus
- [ ] Chicken pox
- [ ] *Erythema infectiosum*
- [ ] Hepatitis
- [ ] Hepatitis B
- [ ] Measles
- [ ] Mumps
- [ ] Parvovirus B19

Bacterial/mycobacterial infections
- [ ] Brucellosis (3)
- [ ] Cholera
- [ ] *Mycoplasma pneumoniae*
- [ ] Pertussis vaccination
- [ ] Tetanus
- [ ] Toxin-mediated staphylococcal infection
- [ ] Tuberculosis
- [ ] BCG

Other infections
- [ ] Malaria (5)
- [ ] Acquired toxoplasmosis (2)

Infectious Diseases

- [ ] *Pneumocystis carinii*
- [ ] Congenital toxoplasmosis
- [ ] *Giardia lamblia*
- [ ] *Chlamydia trachomatis*

Miscellaneous
- [ ] Antibiotic prophylaxis
- [ ] Cerebral abscess
- [ ] Fever and splenomegaly
- [ ] Epiglottitis
- [ ] Immunisation
- [ ] Infections associated with eosinophilia
- [ ] Infectious causes of hydrops fetalis
- [ ] Tonsillar exudates
- [ ] Kawasaki's disease
- [ ] Post-splenectomy septicaemia

METABOLIC DISEASE: EXAM TOPICS

July 1996
- G6PD deficiency
- Phenylketonuria
- Metabolic acidosis

February 1996
- Causes of acidosis
- Methaemoglobinaemia
- Aldosterone
- 21 hydroxylase deficiency

October 1995
- Wilson's disease
- Congenital adrenal hyperplasia
- Insulin dependent diabetes mellitus
- Methaemoglobinaemia
- Galactosaemia

July 1995
- Gilbert's syndrome
- Treatment of hyperkalaemia
- Homocystinuria
- Phenylketonuria

October 1994
- Calcium metabolism

July 1994
- Enzyme defects associated with body odour

February 1994
- Metabolic acidosis
- Hypoglycaemia

METABOLIC DISEASE: TOPIC FREQUENCY INDEX

Metabolic acidosis	July 1996, Feb 1994
Methaemoglobinaemia	Feb 1996, Oct 1995
Phenylketonuria	July 1996, July 1995
21 hydroxylase deficiency	Feb 1996
Aldosterone	Feb 1996
Calcium metabolism	Oct 1994
Causes of acidosis	Feb 1996
Congenital adrenal hyperplasia	Oct 1995
Enzyme defects associated with body odour	July 1994
G6PD deficiency	July 1996
Galactosaemia	Oct 1995
Gilbert's syndrome	July 1995
Homocystinuria	July 1995
Hypoglycaemia	Feb 1994
Treatment of hyperkalaemia	July 1995
Wilson's disease	Oct 1995

METABOLIC DISEASE: REVISION CHECKLIST

Two or three metabolic questions appear in each exam. Numbers in brackets indicate the relative frequency of topics.

Acid/base and electrolytes
- [ ] Metabolic acidosis (2)
- [ ] Causes of acidosis

Inherited metabolic disorders
- [ ] Phenylketonuria (2)
- [ ] 21 hydroxylase deficiency
- [ ] Congenital adrenal hyperplasia
- [ ] G6PD deficiency
- [ ] Galactosaemia
- [ ] Gilbert's syndrome
- [ ] Homocystinuria
- [ ] Wilson's disease

Miscellaneous
- [ ] Methaemoglobinaemia (2)
- [ ] Aldosterone
- [ ] Calcium metabolism
- [ ] Enzyme defects associated with body odour
- [ ] Hypoglycaemia
- [ ] Treatment of hyperkalaemia

NEONATOLOGY: EXAM TOPICS

July 1996
- Respiratory distress
- Breast feeding advantages in pre-term infants
- Convulsions in first week of life

February 1996
- Intrauterine growth retardation complications

October 1995
- Necrotising enterocolitis

July 1995
- Maternal conditions affecting the newborn

February 1995
- Neonatal reflexes
- Increased respiratory rate
- Markers of neonatal infection

October 1994
- Haematological indices at 48 hours of life
- Causes of goitre
- Convulsions
- Prolonged jaundice

July 1994
- Cyanotic heart disease
- Hypoglycaemia
- ABO incompatibility
- Respiratory distress

Neonatology

February 1994
- Convulsions
- Necrotising enterocolitis
- Hypotonia
- Signs of sepsis
- Temperature regulation
- Low birth weight infants
- Birth asphyxia

October 1993
- Maternal conditions affecting the newborn
- Bile stained vomiting
- Clotting abnormalities
- Newborn tachypnoea
- Neonatal emergencies
- Jaundice
- Kernicterus

NEONATOLOGY: TOPIC FREQUENCY INDEX

Respiratory distress	July 1996, Feb 1995, July 1994, Oct 1993
Convulsions	July 1996, Oct 1994, Feb 1994
Sepsis	Feb 1995, Feb 1994
Maternal conditions affecting the newborn	July 1995, Oct 1993
Necrotising enterocolitis	Oct 1995, Feb 1994
Jaundice	Oct 1994, Oct 1993
ABO incompatibility	July 1994
Bile stained vomiting	Oct 1993
Birth asphyxia	Feb 1994
Breast feeding advantages in pre-term infants	July 1996
Causes of goitre	Oct 1994
Clotting abnormalities	Oct 1993
Cyanotic heart disease	July 1994
Haematological indices at 48 hours of life	Oct 1994
Hypoglycaemia	July 1994
Hypotonia	Feb 1994
Intrauterine growth retardation complications	Feb 1996
Kernicterus	Oct 1993
Low birth weight infants	Feb 1994
Neonatal emergencies	Oct 1993
Neonatal reflexes	Feb 1995
Temperature regulation	Feb 1994

NEONATOLOGY: REVISION CHECKLIST

An average of three neonatal questions appear in each exam. Numbers in brackets indicate the relative frequency of topics.

Haematology
- [ ] ABO incompatibility
- [ ] Clotting abnormalities
- [ ] Haematological indices at 48 hours of life
- [ ] Kernicterus

Cardio-respiratory
- [ ] Respiratory distress (4)
- [ ] Cyanotic heart disease

Low birth weight and prematurity
- [ ] Breast feeding advantages in pre-term infants
- [ ] Low birth weight infants
- [ ] Temperature regulation
- [ ] Hypoglycaemia
- [ ] Intrauterine growth retardation complications

Neurology
- [ ] Convulsions (3)
- [ ] Birth asphyxia
- [ ] Hypotonia
- [ ] Neonatal reflexes

Gastroenterology
- [ ] Necrotising enterocolitis (2)
- [ ] Jaundice (2)
- [ ] Bile stained vomiting

Miscellaneous
- [ ] Sepsis (2)
- [ ] Maternal conditions affecting the newborn (2)
- [ ] Causes of goitre
- [ ] Neonatal emergencies

NEPHROLOGY: EXAM TOPICS

July 1996
    End-stage renal failure
    Henoch-Schönlein purpura
    Circumcision: medical indications

February 1996
    Nephrotic syndrome

October 1995
    Urinary tract infection
    Membranous glomerulonephritis
    Type I renal tubular acidosis

July 1995
    Macroscopic haematuria
    Minimal change glomerulonephritis

February 1995
    Haemolytic uraemic syndrome
    Hypertension

October 1994
    Distal Type IV renal tubular acidosis
    Nephrotic syndrome
    Renal failure

July 1994
    Urinary tract infection
    Minimal change glomerulonephritis
    Chronic renal failure

February 1994
    Nephrotic syndrome
    Haemolytic uraemic syndrome

Nephrology

Uraemic osteodystrophy

October 1993
Circumcision: medical indications

NEPHROLOGY: TOPIC FREQUENCY INDEX	
Nephrotic syndrome	Feb 1996, Oct 1994, Feb 1994
Chronic renal failure	July 1996, July 1994
Circumcision: medical indications	July 1996, Oct 1993
Renal tubular acidosis	Oct 1995, Oct 1994
Haemolytic uraemic syndrome	Feb 1995, Feb 1994
Minimal change glomerulonephritis	July 1995, July 1994
Urinary tract infection	Oct 1995, July 1994
Henoch-Schönlein purpura	July 1996
Hypertension	Feb 1995
Macroscopic haematuria	July 1995
Membranous glomerulonephritis	Oct 1995
Renal failure	Oct 1994
Uraemic osteodystrophy	Feb 1994

NEPHROLOGY: REVISION CHECKLIST

An average of three questions appear in each exam. Numbers in brackets indicate the relative frequency of topics.

Renal failure
- [ ] Chronic renal failure (2)
- [ ] Renal failure
- [ ] Uraemic osteodystrophy

Nephrotic/nephritic syndromes
- [ ] Nephrotic syndrome (3)
- [ ] Minimal change glomerulonephritis (2)
- [ ] Membrane glomerulonephritis

Urinary abnormalities
- [ ] Urinary tract infection (2)
- [ ] Macroscopic haematuria

Miscellaneous
- [ ] Circumcision: medical indications (2)
- [ ] Renal tubular acidosis (2)
- [ ] Haemolytic uraemic syndrome (2)
- [ ] Henoch-Schönlein purpura
- [ ] Hypertension

NEUROLOGY: EXAM TOPICS

July 1996
- Parinaud's syndrome
- Right homonymous hemianopia
- Infant hypotonia
- Epilepsy

February 1996
- Posterior interosseus nerve
- Duchenne muscular dystrophy
- Temporal lobe epilepsy
- Cranial nerves
- Febrile convulsions

October 1995
- Duchenne muscular dystrophy
- Spinal cord lesions
- Petit mal epilepsy
- Guillain-Barré syndrome
- Median nerve

July 1995
- Cortico-spinal tracts
- Downbeat nystagmus
- Radial nerve trauma
- Acute encephalitis
- Night time seizures

February 1995
- Prefrontal cortex lesions
- Lumbar punctures
- Vertigo
- Partial complex seizures
- Childhood facial palsy

Neurology

October 1994
    Reflexes in a 6-month-old
    Grimacing in an eleven-year-old
    Papilloedema
    Complete unilateral facial hemiparesis
    Hemiplegic migraine
    Control of finger movements
    Third nerve palsy

July 1994
    Hypotonia
    Benign Rolandic epilepsy
    Parietal lobe lesions
    6th nerve palsy
    Pupillary light reflex
    Truncal ataxia

February 1994
    Childhood stroke
    Intranuclear ophthalmoplegia
    Myotonic dystrophy
    Head injury
    Spinal cord anatomy

October 1993
    Innervation of the hand

NEUROLOGY: TOPIC FREQUENCY INDEX

Duchenne muscular dystrophy	Feb 1996, Oct 1995
Hypotonia	July 1996, July 1994
6th nerve palsy	July 1994
Acute encephalitis	July 1995
Benign Rolandic epilepsy	July 1994
Childhood facial palsy	Feb 1995
Childhood stroke	Feb 1994
Complete unilateral facial hemiparesis	Oct 1994
Control of finger movements	Oct 1994
Cortico-spinal tracts	July 1995
Cranial nerves	Feb 1996
Downbeat nystagmus	July 1995
Epilepsy	July 1996
Febrile convulsions	Feb 1996
Grimacing in an eleven-year-old	Oct 1994
Guillain-Barré syndrome	Oct 1995
Head injury	Feb 1994
Hemiplegic migraine	Oct 1994
Innervation of the hand	Oct 1993
Intranuclear ophthalmoplegia	Feb 1994
Lumbar punctures	Feb 1995
Median nerve	Oct 1995
Myotonic dystrophy	Feb 1994
Night time seizures	July 1995
Papilloedema	Oct 1994
Parinaud's syndrome	July 1996
Parietal lobe lesions	July 1994
Partial complex seizures	Feb 1995
Petit mal epilepsy	Oct 1995
Posterior interosseus nerve	Feb 1996
Prefrontal cortex lesions	Feb 1995
Pupillary light reflex	July 1994
Radial nerve trauma	July 1995

Neurology

Reflexes in a 6-month-old	Oct 1994
Right homonymous hemianopia	July 1996
Spinal cord anatomy	Feb 1994
Spinal cord lesions	Oct 1995
Temporal lobe epilepsy	Feb 1996
Third nerve palsy	Oct 1994
Truncal ataxia	July 1994
Vertigo	Feb 1995

NEUROLOGY: REVISION CHECKLIST

Neurology questions are consistently the most frequently asked in the exam. An average of over five questions appear in each exam although these will often be part of questions relevant to other specialties such as neonatology. Note that questions relating to the developmental milestones have been included in the section on growth and development. Numbers in brackets indicate the relative frequency of topics.

Brain and cerebral circulation
- [ ] Acute encephalitis
- [ ] Childhood stroke
- [ ] Febrile convulsions
- [ ] Head injury
- [ ] Papilloedema
- [ ] Parinaud's syndrome
- [ ] Parietal lobe lesions
- [ ] Prefrontal cortex lesions

Epilepsy
- [ ] Temporal lobe epilepsy
- [ ] Partial complex seizures
- [ ] Petit mal epilepsy
- [ ] Night time seizures
- [ ] Benign Rolandic epilepsy
- [ ] Epilepsy

Cord and peripheral nerve
- [ ] Control of finger movements
- [ ] Cortico-spinal tracts
- [ ] Guillain-Barré syndrome
- [ ] Innervation of the hand
- [ ] Median nerve
- [ ] Posterior interosseus nerve

- ☐ Radial nerve trauma
- ☐ Spinal cord anatomy
- ☐ Spinal cord lesions

Cranial nerve
- ☐ Third nerve palsy
- ☐ 6th nerve palsy
- ☐ Childhood facial palsy
- ☐ Complete unilateral facial hemiparesis
- ☐ Cranial nerves
- ☐ Intranuclear ophthalmoplegia
- ☐ Pupillary light reflex
- ☐ Right homonymous hemianopia

Miscellaneous
- ☐ Hypotonia (2)
- ☐ Duchenne muscular dystrophy (2)
- ☐ Downbeat nystagmus
- ☐ Grimacing in an eleven-year-old
- ☐ Hemiplegic migraine
- ☐ Reflexes in a 6-month-old
- ☐ Lumbar punctures
- ☐ Truncal ataxia
- ☐ Myotonic dystrophy
- ☐ Vertigo

NUTRITION: EXAM TOPICS

Questions on nutrition are occasionally asked and have been grouped separately from gastroenterology questions.

October 1995
  Protein energy malnutrition

October 1994
  Contraindications to breastfeeding

July 1994
  Human and cows' milk properties

February 1994
  Nutritional requirements of a one-year-old

October 1993
  Breast milk contents

OPHTHALMOLOGY: EXAM TOPICS

Ophthalmology questions appear from time to time and are listed below. Questions on squint, amblyopia and corneal opacities appear most frequently.

February 1996
 Common ophthalmological conditions

October 1995
 Cataracts

July 1995
 Corneal opacities

February 1995
 Central retinal vein occlusion

October 1994
 Convergent squint

PHARMACOLOGY: EXAM TOPICS

July 1996
- Asthma prevention
- Cimetidine
- Theophylline overdose

February 1996
- Gentamicin toxicity
- Drugs in breast milk
- Aminoglycoside toxicity in neonates

October 1995
- Renal failure: contraindications
- Oral contraception and pulmonary embolus

July 1995
- Aspirin overdose
- Steroid withdrawal in children

February 1995
- Drug interactions
- AZT
- Tricyclic antidepressant overdose
- Drugs in renal disease

October 1994
- Antipyretics in infancy
- Sumitriptan
- Paracetamol overdose

July 1994
- Sodium valproate

Pharmacology

February 1994
- Drugs causing acute renal failure
- Gentamicin therapy
- Analgesia
- Anticonvulsants

October 1993
- Side effects of substance abuse
- Phenobarbitone overdose
- Interactions with oral contraceptives
- Poisoning

PHARMACOLOGY: TOPIC FREQUENCY INDEX

Gentamicin therapy and toxicity	Feb 1996, Feb 1994
Oral contraceptives	Oct 1995, Oct 1993
Aminoglycoside toxicity in neonates	Feb 1996
Analgesia	Feb 1994
Anticonvulsants	Feb 1994
Antipyretics in infancy	Oct 1994
Aspirin overdose	July 1995
Asthma prevention	July 1996
AZT	Feb 1995
Cimetidine	July 1996
Drug interactions	Feb 1995
Drugs causing acute renal failure	Feb 1994
Drugs in breast milk	Feb 1996
Drugs in renal disease	Feb 1995
Paracetamol overdose	Oct 1994
Phenobarbitone overdose	Oct 1993
Poisoning	Oct 1993
Renal failure: contraindications	Oct 1995
Side effects of substance abuse	Oct 1993
Sodium valproate	July 1994
Steroid withdrawal in children	July 1995
Sumitriptan	Oct 1994
Theophylline overdose	July 1996
Tricyclic antidepressant overdose	Feb 1995

PHARMACOLOGY: REVISION CHECKLIST

An average of two pharmacology questions appear in each exam although stems of non-pharmacological questions may often contain an option relevant to pharmacology. Numbers in brackets indicate the relative frequency of topics.

Drug overdose or abuse
- [ ] Aspirin overdose
- [ ] Theophylline overdose
- [ ] Tricyclic antidepressant overdose
- [ ] Paracetamol overdose
- [ ] Phenobarbitone overdose

Toxicity
- [ ] Gentamicin therapy and toxicity (2)
- [ ] Aminoglycoside toxicity in neonates
- [ ] Drug interactions
- [ ] Drugs causing acute renal failure
- [ ] Poisoning
- [ ] Renal failure: contraindications
- [ ] Side effects of substance abuse

Individual drugs
- [ ] AZT
- [ ] Cimetidine
- [ ] Sodium valproate
- [ ] Steroid withdrawal in children
- [ ] Sumitriptan

Classes of drugs
- [ ] Oral contraceptives (2)
- [ ] Analgesia
- [ ] Anticonvulsants
- [ ] Antipyretics in infancy
- [ ] Asthma prevention

Miscellaneous
- [ ] Drugs in breast milk
- [ ] Drugs in renal disease

PSYCHIATRY: EXAM TOPICS

July 1996
- Obsessive disorders
- Schizophrenia

February 1996
- Schizophrenia
- Somatisation

October 1995
- Sexual abuse
- Prevalence of psychiatric disorders
- Abdominal pain
- Bulimia nervosa

July 1995
- Autism
- General reasons for referral
- Anorexia nervosa

February 1995
- Schizophrenia
- Anorexia nervosa
- School refusal
- Munchausen's by proxy
- Attention deficit disorders

October 1994
- Sexual abuse
- Causes for referral of a 5-year-old

Psychiatry

July 1994
- School refusal
- Autism
- Attention deficit disorders
- Child abuse

February 1994
- Symptoms of anxiety

October 1993
- Sexual abuse
- Attention deficit disorders
- Alcoholism

PSYCHIATRY: TOPIC FREQUENCY INDEX

Attention deficit disorders	Feb 1995, July 1994, Oct 1993
Schizophrenia	July 1996, Feb 1996, Feb 1995
Sexual abuse	Oct 1995, Oct 1994, Oct 1993
Anorexia nervosa	July 1995, Feb 1995
Autism	July 1995, July 1994
School refusal	Feb 1995, July 1994
Abdominal pain	Oct 1995
Alcoholism	Oct 1993
Bulimia nervosa	Oct 1995
Causes for referral of a 5-year-old	Oct 1994
Child abuse	July 1994
General reasons for referral	July 1995
Munchausen's by proxy	Feb 1995
Obsessive disorders	July 1996
Prevalence of psychiatric disorders	Oct 1995
Somatisation	Feb 1996
Symptoms of anxiety	Feb 1994

PSYCHIATRY: REVISION CHECKLIST

An average of three questions appear in each exam. Numbers in brackets indicate the relative frequency of topics.

Paediatric psychiatry
- [ ] Attention deficit disorders (3)
- [ ] Sexual abuse (3)
- [ ] Autism (2)
- [ ] School refusal (2)
- [ ] Abdominal pain
- [ ] Causes for referral of a 5-year-old
- [ ] Child abuse
- [ ] General reasons for referral
- [ ] Munchausen's by proxy

Psychotic illness
- [ ] Schizophrenia (3)

Eating disorders
- [ ] Anorexia nervosa (2)
- [ ] Bulimia nervosa

Miscellaneous
- [ ] Alcoholism
- [ ] Prevalence of psychiatric disorders
- [ ] Somatisation
- [ ] Obsessive disorders
- [ ] Symptoms of anxiety

RESPIRATORY DISEASE: EXAM TOPICS

July 1996
- Sweat test
- Bronchiectasis
- Teenage asthma
- Breath-holding spells

February 1996
- Bronchiolitis
- Pneumothorax
- Cystic fibrosis
- Sleep apnoea
- Pneumonia

October 1995
- Bronchoconstriction
- Bronchopulmonary dysplasia
- Bronchiolitis
- Cystic fibrosis

July 1995
- Exercise-induced asthma
- Cystic fibrosis

February 1995
- Community acquired pneumonia
- Sleep apnoea
- Asthma

October 1994
- Cystic fibrosis
- Hypoxaemic respiratory failure

July 1994
- Asthma
- Croup

Respiratory Disease

February 1994
　　Surfactant
　　Pulmonary function
　　Pulmonary cavitation

October 1993
　　Cystic fibrosis
　　Plethoric lung fields
　　Crackles at lung bases
　　Bronchiectasis

RESPIRATORY DISEASE: TOPIC FREQUENCY INDEX

Cystic fibrosis	Feb 1996, Oct 1995, July 1995, Oct 1994, Oct 1993
Asthma	July 1996, July 1995, Feb 1995, July 1994
Bronchiectasis	July 1996, Oct 1993
Bronchiolitis	Feb 1996, Oct 1995
Sleep apnoea	Feb 1996, Feb 1995
Breath-holding spells	July 1996
Bronchoconstriction	Oct 1995
Bronchopulmonary dysplasia	Oct 1995
Community acquired pneumonia	Feb 1995
Crackles at lung bases	Oct 1993
Croup	July 1994
Hypoxaemic respiratory failure	Oct 1994
Plethoric lung fields	Oct 1993
Pneumonia	Feb 1996
Pneumothorax	Feb 1996
Pulmonary cavitation	Feb 1994
Pulmonary function	Feb 1994
Surfactant	Feb 1994
Sweat test	July 1996

RESPIRATORY DISEASE: REVISION CHECKLIST

An average of four questions appear in each exam. Numbers in brackets indicate the relative frequency of topics.

Infection
- [ ] Bronchiolitis (2)
- [ ] Community acquired pneumonia
- [ ] Crackles at lung bases
- [ ] Croup
- [ ] Pneumonia
- [ ] Pulmonary cavitation

Reversible/non-reversible lung disease
- [ ] Cystic fibrosis (5)
- [ ] Asthma (4)
- [ ] Bronchiectasis (2)
- [ ] Bronchoconstriction
- [ ] Bronchopulmonary dysplasia

Physiology
- [ ] Pulmonary function

Miscellaneous
- [ ] Sleep apnoea (2)
- [ ] Breath-holding spells
- [ ] Hypoxaemic respiratory failure
- [ ] Plethoric lung fields
- [ ] Pneumothorax
- [ ] Surfactant
- [ ] Sweat test

RHEUMATOLOGY: EXAM TOPICS

Most examinations will contain at least one question relating to rheumatology. Questions are usually relevant to paediatrics and rarely purely adult orientated.

July 1996
    Juvenile chronic arthritis

October 1995
    Systemic lupus erythematosus

July 1995
    Behçet's disease

February 1995
    Rheumatoid arthritis
    Swollen joints in childhood

July 1994
    Polyarthritis

February 1994
    Rheumatoid arthritis

October 1993
    Systemic lupus erythematosus

STATISTICS: EXAM TOPICS

All the examinations thus far have contained one pure statistics question. The topics are indicated below.

July 1996
    2x2 table

February 1996
    Normal distribution

October 1995
    Standard deviation

July 1995
    Correlation coefficients and p values

February 1995
    Significance tests

October 1994
    Normal distribution

July 1994
    Tests of significance

February 1994
    Skewed distributions, means and medians

October 1993
    Tests of significance

MCQ PRACTICE EXAMINATION

The following Practice Examination was compiled from questions remembered by candidates who sat the MRCP Part 1 Paediatric examination. The questions are thus similar to those that have appeared in the actual College examination. The examination has been structured in such a way that the relative distribution of topics reflects that set by the College (see Foreword page v). The answers have been provided by experienced PasTest lecturers although, as with all multiple choice questions, both the questions and the answers may be open to interpretation.

Mark your answers with a tick, cross or question mark in the boxes provided.

NEUROLOGY

1. **Concerning Duchenne muscular dystrophy**

   - A the brothers of 50% of affected individuals will be affected
   - B myotonia is absent
   - C it may be associated with walking late
   - D ankle reflexes remain until late
   - E a high CPK in a sister of an affected individual suggests that she may be a carrier

2. **In acute encephalitis**

   - A epilepsy is a recognised sequelae
   - B herpes simplex is the commonest cause of sporadic viral encephalitis in the UK
   - C abnormal EEG changes may be present early in the disease even if the CT scan is normal
   - D acyclovir is an effective treatment for herpes simplex
   - E absence of pleocytosis in the CSF excludes the diagnosis

3. **Regarding the cortico-spinal (pyramidal) tracts**

   - A 50% originate in the post central gyrus
   - B three quarters cross at the medulla
   - C lesions only affect proximal regions of limbs
   - D the motor cortex is activated before initiation of movement
   - E they are fast conducting tracts

MCQ Practice Examination

4. **Down beat nystagmus is a feature of**

   - [ ] A Type I Chiari malformation
   - [ ] B dysgerminoma
   - [ ] C phenytoin toxicity
   - [ ] D aqueduct stenosis
   - [ ] E lesion of medial longitudinal fasciculus

5. **The following findings exclude a diagnosis of Guillain-Barré syndrome:**

   - [ ] A a normal CSF
   - [ ] B an ophthalmoplegia
   - [ ] C autonomic failure
   - [ ] D a sensory level at D10
   - [ ] E muscle wasting

INFECTIOUS DISEASES

6. **An infant is more likely to acquire HIV from an HIV-positive mother if**

   - [ ] A born by Caesarian section
   - [ ] B immunised with diphtheria, tetanus and polio immunisation
   - [ ] C breast fed
   - [ ] D the mother has a low CD4 count
   - [ ] E immunised with haemophilus influenzae type b vaccine

7. **Regarding malaria**

   - [ ] A *Plasmodium falciparum* does not have an exoerythrocytic cycle
   - [ ] B blood glucose may be increased in cerebral malaria
   - [ ] C merozoites do not re-infect the liver
   - [ ] D it is transmitted by sporozoites carried by mosquitoes
   - [ ] E *P. vivax* preferentially infect old red blood cells

MCQ Practice Examination

8. Recognised features of brucellosis include

   ☐ A epididymo-orchitis
   ☐ B cranial nerve palsies
   ☐ C vesicular eruption
   ☐ D positive Weil-Felix test
   ☐ E leucocytosis

9. Concerning Epstein-Barr virus (EBV) (infectious mononucleosis)

   ☐ A the presence of petechiae between the hard and soft palate supports the diagnosis
   ☐ B typically a rash occurs following intravenous administration of penicillin
   ☐ C Guillain-Barré syndrome is a recognised sequelae
   ☐ D hepatitis is common
   ☐ E cervical lymphadenopathy and splenomegaly are due to extreme B cell hyperactivity

10. Regarding rubella

    ☐ A the incubation period is 7 to 10 days
    ☐ B it is associated with arthritis
    ☐ C abortion should be offered to those who become infected in the first two months of pregnancy
    ☐ D it can cause idiopathic thrombocytopenic purpura
    ☐ E it shows splenomegaly more than infectious mononucleosis

CARDIOLOGY

11. In the Wolff-Parkinson-White syndrome

    ☐ A the accessory pathway connects the atrial and ventricular myocardium
    ☐ B junctional tachycardias are more commonly broad than narrow complex
    ☐ C narrow complex tachycardia is usually regular
    ☐ D verapamil is the drug of choice for the control of atrial fibrillation
    ☐ E amiodarone prolongs the refractory period (recovery time) in the accessory pathway

MCQ Practice Examination

12. In ostium secundum septal defects

- [ ] A over 10% close spontaneously
- [ ] B they frequently present as AF in middle age
- [ ] C they cannot be diagnosed on trans-oesophageal echocardiography
- [ ] D they rarely lead to pulmonary hypertension in childhood
- [ ] E they are more apparent clinically than pulmonary stenosis

13. A 2-day-old neonate with cyanotic congenital heart disease

- [ ] A is likely to have a left to right shunt
- [ ] B will benefit from indomethacin
- [ ] C the most likely diagnosis is total anomalous pulmonary venous D
- [ ] D it is likely that detailed cardiac examination will be normal
- [ ] E may have Ebstein's anomaly

14. A heart murmur in a 5-year-old child is more likely to have a structural cardiac lesion underlying it if

- [ ] A the murmur changes when position is changed
- [ ] B the murmur is heard only in the neck
- [ ] C it is associated with a second heart sound widely split on inspiration
- [ ] D the murmur is diastolic
- [ ] E there is a palpable thrill

15. Cannon waves are a recognised feature of

- [ ] A junctional (A-V nodal) rhythm
- [ ] B complete heart block
- [ ] C ventricular tachycardia
- [ ] D hypertrophic cardiomyopathy with obstruction
- [ ] E pulmonary stenosis

MCQ Practice Examination

RESPIRATORY

16. Cystic fibrosis may present in the following ways:

- [ ] A nasal polyps
- [ ] B rectal prolapse
- [ ] C circulatory collapse in hot weather
- [ ] D intestinal obstruction in neonatal period
- [ ] E mental retardation

17. Exercise-induced asthma

- [ ] A can be reliably diagnosed in the 6 minute exercise test
- [ ] B has an increased likelihood of repeat attack up to 45 minutes after the first attack
- [ ] C can be prevented by taking corticosteroids prior to exercise
- [ ] D causes release of inflammatory mediators
- [ ] E has no inflammatory component

18. Acute bronchiolitis is

- [ ] A more common in children of between 18 months and 36 months of age
- [ ] B more serious in patients with bronchopulmonary dysplasia
- [ ] C caused by respiratory synctial virus
- [ ] D associated with hyperexpanded rib cage in the acute phase
- [ ] E a recognised cause of bronchiectasis

19. Recognised features of sleep apnoea syndrome include

- [ ] A apnoeas longest during non-rapid eye movement sleep
- [ ] B morning headache
- [ ] C rapid eye movement (REM) sleep within 10 minutes of sleep onset
- [ ] D daytime somnolence
- [ ] E recurrent tachycardia during apnoeas

MCQ Practice Examination

HAEMATOLOGY/ONCOLOGY

20. Recognised features of ABO incompatibility include

- [ ] A   normal haemoglobin on day 1
- [ ] B   worsening with subsequent pregnancies
- [ ] C   conjugated hyperbilirubinaemia
- [ ] D   negative Coombs' test
- [ ] E   may occur in first pregnancy

21. The following are causes of reticulocyte count over 10%:

- [ ] A   rhesus incompatibility
- [ ] B   parvovirus
- [ ] C   aplastic anaemia
- [ ] D   sickle cell disease
- [ ] E   Fanconi anaemia

22. A prolonged bleeding time is a characteristic of

- [ ] A   haemophilia
- [ ] B   idiopathic thrombocytopenic purpura
- [ ] C   Christmas disease
- [ ] D   Henoch-Schönlein purpura
- [ ] E   von Willebrand's disease

23. The following are more common in children with Wilm's tumours compared with an age-matched normal population:

- [ ] A   Beckwith Wiederman syndrome
- [ ] B   hemihypertrophy
- [ ] C   familiar aniridia
- [ ] D   reaction to DPT vaccination
- [ ] E   genitourinary abnormalities

MCQ Practice Examination

GROWTH AND DEVELOPMENT

24. A child of 12 months would be expected to

- [ ] A build a tower of 3 cubes
- [ ] B speak 5 words in context
- [ ] C remove a garment of clothing
- [ ] D feed him/herself with a spoon
- [ ] E walk around a cot

25. In a child aged 9 months a large head may be due to

- [ ] A achondroplasia
- [ ] B genetic predisposition
- [ ] C craniosynostosis
- [ ] D hydrocephalus
- [ ] E failure to thrive

26. Delayed bone age is seen with

- [ ] A partially treated congenital adrenal hyperplasia
- [ ] B Turner's syndrome
- [ ] C growth hormone insufficiency
- [ ] D simple obesity
- [ ] E social deprivation

PSYCHIATRY

27. Anorexia nervosa

- [ ] A does not occur in males
- [ ] B has no increased incidence of suicide
- [ ] C reduces anxiety
- [ ] D may be associated with purgative abuse
- [ ] E is associated with loss of hair

MCQ Practice Examination

28. Characteristics of schizophrenia include

- [ ] A grossly disorganised behaviour
- [ ] B delusions of control
- [ ] C intellectual capacity usually maintained
- [ ] D incongruity of mood
- [ ] E visual hallucinations

29. Autism is associated with

- [ ] A females
- [ ] B decreased eye contact
- [ ] C obsessional behaviour
- [ ] D delay in language development
- [ ] E social deprivation

NEONATOLOGY

30. Maternal conditions that may affect the newborn child include

- [ ] A phenylketonuria
- [ ] B maternal diabetes
- [ ] C multiple sclerosis
- [ ] D anticoagulant ingestion during pregnancy
- [ ] E idiopathic thrombocytopenic purpura (ITP)

31. Features predisposing to NEC in the neonatal period include

- [ ] A polycythaemia
- [ ] B asphyxia
- [ ] C umbilical artery catheter
- [ ] D maternal Crohn's disease
- [ ] E Hirschsprung's disease

MCQ Practice Examination

32. **The following are more likely to occur in a baby with intrauterine growth retardation:**

- [ ] A respiratory distress syndrome
- [ ] B hypothermia
- [ ] C polycythaemia
- [ ] D birth asphyxia
- [ ] E hypoglycaemia

GASTROENTEROLOGY

33. **Causes of bloody diarrhoea in childhood include**

- [ ] A verotoxin producing *E. coli*
- [ ] B *Campylobacter jejuni*
- [ ] C *Cryptosporidium*
- [ ] D *Giardia*
- [ ] E rotavirus

34. **In an otherwise well and thriving child with recurrent abdominal pain**

- [ ] A there is an underlying organic problem in under 10% of cases
- [ ] B pain away from the periumbilical area suggests an underlying cause to be more likely
- [ ] C an upper oesophagogastroscopy should be performed
- [ ] D the pain will respond to a low residue diet
- [ ] E rectal examination should be performed

35. **The following may be features of ulcerative colitis:**

- [ ] A short stature
- [ ] B polyarthritis
- [ ] C irritability
- [ ] D polycythaemia
- [ ] E clubbing

ENDOCRINOLOGY

36. A 15-year-old girl suffers from loss of weight and amenorrhoea. The following are consistent with a diagnosis of anorexia:

- [ ] A buccal pigmentation
- [ ] B eating binges
- [ ] C high luteinising hormone
- [ ] D excessive exercising
- [ ] E hypokalaemia

37. Calcitonin

- [ ] A secretion is increased by a fall in serum calcium concentration
- [ ] B inhibits bone resorption
- [ ] C is a single chain polypeptide
- [ ] D is secreted in excess in patients with medullary carcinoma of the thyroid
- [ ] E is secreted by the thyroid epithelial cells

38. There are raised parathyroid hormone levels in

- [ ] A pseudohypoparathyroidism
- [ ] B vitamin D dependent rickets
- [ ] C Paget's disease
- [ ] D chronic renal failure
- [ ] E multiple myeloma

IMMUNOLOGY

39. The following contribute to the natural immunity transmitted in breast milk:

- [ ] A macrophages
- [ ] B natural killer cells
- [ ] C lactoterria
- [ ] D mast cells
- [ ] E secretory IgA

MCQ Practice Examination

40. Complement plays a role in the following:

- [ ] A paroxysmal nocturnal haematuria
- [ ] B systemic lupus erythematosus (SLE)
- [ ] C extrinsic allergic alveolitis
- [ ] D sarcoidosis
- [ ] E post streptococcal glomerulonephritis (PSGN)

41. The following is true of childhood immunisations:

- [ ] A egg protein intolerance is an absolute contraindication to MMR
- [ ] B a family history of epilepsy is a contraindication
- [ ] C it is safe to give children with immunodeficiency varicella vaccine
- [ ] D when giving the oral polio vaccine, breast feeding should be suspended
- [ ] E chicken pox vaccination is safe in a child with malignancy

NEPHROLOGY

42. In a 10-year-old girl who presents with sudden onset of facial oedema and smoky urine 10 days after a sore throat

- [ ] A the CXR may show bat wing shadowing
- [ ] B a BP of 140/100 would suggest a diagnosis of nephrotic syndrome
- [ ] C diuretics are contraindicated in the acute phase
- [ ] D steroids should start on day 3
- [ ] E complement levels will be decreased

43. Type I renal tubular acidosis

- [ ] A only occurs in children
- [ ] B is caused by a failure of hydrores ion secretion
- [ ] C is associated with renal calcification
- [ ] D typically leads to hypovolaemia
- [ ] E characteristically involves a failure to acidify urine below pH 7

MCQ Practice Examination

44. The following are characteristic of minimal change glomerulonephritis:

- [ ] A IgG deposited in kidney
- [ ] B selective proteinuria
- [ ] C diastolic hypertension between relapses
- [ ] D chronic renal failure
- [ ] E response to steroids within four weeks of treatment

GENERAL PAEDIATRICS

45. The sudden onset of acute painful scrotal swelling may be caused by

- [ ] A torsion of the appendix of the testis
- [ ] B incarcerated hernia
- [ ] C Henoch-Schönlein syndrome
- [ ] D leukaemia
- [ ] E idiopathic scrotal oedema

46. Decreased neck mobility is found in

- [ ] A Down's syndrome
- [ ] B cerebellar medulloblastoma
- [ ] C acute poliomyelitis
- [ ] D Still's disease
- [ ] E muscular dystrophy

PHARMACOLOGY

47. The following may result in renal dysfunction in a neonate treated with gentamicin:

- [ ] A hypokalaemia
- [ ] B frusemide
- [ ] C cephalosporins
- [ ] D birth asphyxia
- [ ] E concomittant use of amphotericin B

MCQ Practice Examination

48. **Pulmonary embolism in those taking the combined (oestrogen plus progestogen) oral contraceptive pill**

- [ ] A is causally related to the progestogen component
- [ ] B is more likely to occur in the presence of antithrombin III deficiency
- [ ] C is more likely to occur in the presence of protein C deficiency
- [ ] D is an absolute contraindication to further combined oral contraceptive treatment
- [ ] E is more likely to occur in cigarette smokers than non-smokers

INBORN ERRORS OF METABOLISM

49. **Concerning insulin dependent diabetes mellitus in children**

- [ ] A microangiopathic changes are rare before puberty
- [ ] B isophane is shorter acting than soluble insulin
- [ ] C lipohypertrophy is more common than lipoatrophy
- [ ] D fructosamine can be used to monitor glucose control
- [ ] E insulin requirements increase after diagnosis

50. **The following are consistent with untreated 21 hydroxylase deficiency:**

- [ ] A high ACTH
- [ ] B increased renin
- [ ] C high levels of 17 hydroxyprogesterone
- [ ] D low sodium
- [ ] E increased aldosterone

MCQ Practice Examination

GENETICS

51. The following are transmitted as autosomal dominant traits:

- [ ] A congenital spherocytosis
- [ ] B vitamin D resistant rickets
- [ ] C congenital adrenal hyperplasia
- [ ] D hereditary haemorrhagic telangiectasia
- [ ] E infantile polycystic kidney disease

52. Fragile X

- [ ] A is associated with macrorchidism
- [ ] B has triple code amplification
- [ ] C has an incidence of 1:10000 in males
- [ ] D results in a decrease in fertility
- [ ] E is found only in males

EMBRYOLOGY

53. In embryology

- [ ] A most defects occur as a result of exposure to teratogens in the first 2 weeks post conception
- [ ] B the urachus becomes the median umbilical ligament
- [ ] C the mesonephric duct becomes the female organs
- [ ] D the thyroid develops from the floor of the primitive larynx
- [ ] E melanocytes originate from neural crest cells

NUTRITION

54. Recognised associations of protein energy malnutrition include

- [ ] A albumin is typically low
- [ ] B increased levels of free T3
- [ ] C increased reaction to tuberculin testing
- [ ] D fatty liver
- [ ] E increased levels of IgE

MCQ Practice Examination

OPHTHALMOLOGY

55. Concerning ophthalmology

- [ ] A a 3 month child with a squint should be referred for indirect ophthalmoscopy
- [ ] B a cover test detects amblyopia
- [ ] C a child with visual impairment and no glasses is unable to go to school
- [ ] D myopia is commonly caused by retrolental fibroplasia
- [ ] E a child with diminished visual acuity can be left without treatment until school entrance

RHEUMATOLOGY

56. Concerning systemic lupus erythematosus (SLE)

- [ ] A antibodies against double-stranded DNA are a typical finding
- [ ] B haematoxylin bodies occur in areas of inflammation
- [ ] C it usually progresses to renal failure within two years
- [ ] D deposition of complement component C3 occurs in the glomerular basement membrane
- [ ] E polymorphonuclear leucocytosis is a recognised feature

STATISTICS

57. If a characteristic is normally distributed in a population

- [ ] A the median value will be less than the mean
- [ ] B the modal value will be identical with the mean
- [ ] C there will be equal numbers who have more or less of the characteristic than the mean
- [ ] D 20% of the individuals will be beyond two standard deviations from the mean
- [ ] E this implies that most of the population are normal individuals

MCQ Practice Examination

SURGERY

58. The following are true of umbilical hernia:

- ☐ A it is more common in Caucasians than in other races
- ☐ B it is commonly associated with hypothyroidism
- ☐ C it must be operated on before two years of age
- ☐ D it becomes obstructed in 2% of cases
- ☐ E it is more likely to resolve spontaneously if small

EARS, NOSE AND THROAT

59. The following is true regarding serous otitis media in children:

- ☐ A there is increased incidence in children whose parents smoke
- ☐ B it does not resolve spontaneously
- ☐ C it is asymptomatic
- ☐ D it may lead to learning difficulties
- ☐ E breast feeding is protective

MEDIATORS

60. Atrial natriuretic peptide

- ☐ A is secreted in response to a stretch in the right atrium
- ☐ B suppresses aldosterone
- ☐ C is inactivated by neutral endopeptidase
- ☐ D is ionotropic
- ☐ E is a direct vasodilator

PRACTICE EXAM ANSWERS

1. CDE
Duchenne muscular dystrophy is usually inherited as a X-linked disorder, such that the mother is a carrier and her sons that inherit the abnormal X will be affected, and those with the normal X will be normal. Daughters have a 50% chance of being a carrier, this can be determined genetically in an informative family and 60–80% of carriers have elevated levels of CPK. About one-third of cases are new mutations, so that some children may not have an affected sibling. Ankle reflexes are only lost very late on in the disease as the primary problem is that of the musculature, the nervous pathways remain intact.

2. ABCD
The commonest cause of viral encephalitis in the paediatric population is herpes zoster. There may be a normal CSF on initial examination, with little or no pleocytosis and remarkably normal biochemistry. The outcome of encephalitis is very variable, and fits and other neurological sequelae are not uncommon. Characteristic EEG changes are often only present late on in the disease process, but some changes may be present early on, in the presence of a normal CT scan.

3. BD
Fibres of the cortico-spinal tract arise as axons of pyramidal cells situated in the fifth layer of the cerebral cortex. About one-third originate from the primary motor cortex, one-third from the secondary motor cortex and one-third from the parietal zone. Hence, two-thirds arise from the precentral gyrus and one-third from the post central gyrus. The majority of cortico-spinal fibres are myelinated and are small, relatively slow-conducting fibres. The majority of fibres decussate in the medulla, whilst the remainder cross the midline in the spinal cord.

4. ACD
Downbeat nystagmus is accentuated by vertical gaze. It may be produced by sedative drugs (especially phenytoin) but otherwise localizes disease to the medulla of the brainstem (although brainstem disorders more commonly produce horizontal nystagmus). Lesions of the medial longitudinal fasciculus cause impaired convergence and lateral conjugate gaze. If the lesion is in the lower part of

Practice Exam Answers

the tract then the VIth cranial nerve will also be involved and there will be defective abduction, causing horizontal nystagmus.

5. D
Guillain-Barré syndrome is an acute demyelinating polyneuropathy and as such may affect any motor, sensory or autonomic nerve. Normal CSF is found in 50% at presentation (and as such should NEVER exclude the diagnosis), and is never abnormal in 10%. A sensory level is not consistent with the diagnosis.

6. C
Approximately 15% of infants in Europe born to HIV-positive mothers acquire HIV perinatally. Breast feeding is known to increase the risk, as is vaginal, especially instrumental, delivery. However, breast feeding is still recommended in developing countries because of the cost of formula milk and the associated risks of diarrhoeal illness. The risk of transmission of HIV is not increased by vaccination of the mother or child and HIV-positive children should receive a normal vaccination schedule, including oral polio.

7. ACD
Malarial sporozoites are injected into the skin by the female *Anopheles* mosquito. They undergo development in the liver and micromerozoites are liberated into the circulation. In *P. vivax* (and possibly *P. ovale* and *P. malariae* but not *P. falciparum*) a latent exoerythrocytic phase in the liver occurs. *P. falciparum* micromerozoites invade all RBCs (and hence causes the most severe disease), whilst *P. vivax* and *P. ovale* preferentially invade reticulocytes and young RBCs and malariae invades senescent RBCs. Each cycle in RBCs terminates with the rupture of the cell and the release of merozoites into the circulation. Hypoglycaemia is a feature of cerebral malaria.

8. AB
Brucella abortius, *B. Melitensis* and *B. suis* cause granuloma formation throughout all organs of the body, the liver and spleen are most commonly affected. A rash occurs in only 5% of patients and is papular, petechial or erythema nodosum. The Weil-Felix reaction is used to diagnose typhus. Blood cultures are positive in 50% of cases of acute brucellosis, and serological diagnosis based on ELISA is possible. Leucocytosis does not usually occur.

Practice Exam Answers

9. ACD
Palatal petechial haemorrhages occur in 25–60% of cases of infectious mononucleosis but are not diagnostic. A rash may occur after the oral or IV administration of ampicillin, but not penicillin. Cervical lymphadenopathy and splenomegaly are characteristic and mild hepatitis is common, with 10% becoming jaundiced. Other manifestations (e.g. myocarditis, mesenteric adenitis, splenic rupture, encephalitis, meningitis and Guillain-Barré syndrome) are rare. Although EBV can infect and cause the proliferation of B cells, the majority of activated lymphocytes seen in peripheral blood, lymph node and spleen are EBV-specific T cells (especially CD8+, cytotoxic T cells).

10. BCD
The incubation period for rubella is 14–21 days, and individuals are infectious from 7 days before the onset of the rash until 2 weeks afterwards. The risk of severe congenital malformation in the fetus is up to 90% in the first two months of pregnancy, so that if there is a significant suspicion of rubella (inc. IgM) in a pregnant woman in this time it is reasonable to offer termination. Recognised sequelae of rubella include an arthropathy and idiopathic thrombocytopenic purpura.

11. ACE
In Wolff-Parkinson-White syndrome 'the most common tachycardia' is a regular narrow complex one which will usually respond to IV adenosine or verapamil. Atrial fibrillation occurs in about 15% and if the accessory pathway allows 1:1 conduction may lead to VF. Thus, drugs which decrease AV are contraindicated because nodal conduction will encourage conduction down the pathway. Amiodarone is an effective drug at preventing conduction in the accessory pathway.

12. D
ASDs comprise 10% of congenital heart disease, the majority being ostium secundum. 10% or less close spontaneously. They are usually asymptomatic in childhood and present in the third or fourth decade with arrhythmias or cardiac failure, or more rarely in later childhood with decreased exercise tolerance. All ostium secundum defects should therefore be closed during childhood. They can be diagnosed on conventional or trans-oesophageal echocardiography. Although

Practice Exam Answers

ASD and PS may sound very similar, the PS is much more likely to cause symptoms.

13. AE
A cyanotic neonate may have respiratory disease, CNS disease or cardiac disease (or rarely methaemoglobinaemia). The differential diagnosis of cyanotic congenital heart disease at this age includes transposition of the great arteries, pulmonary atresia, severe tetralogy of Fallot, tricuspid atresia with restricted pulmonary blood flow, critical pulmonary stenosis and Ebstein's anomaly of the tricuspid valve. In all of these conditions a left to right shunt is beneficial to the infant to allow the passage of unoxygenated blood in the aorta through the lungs. Indomethacin may therefore be harmful as it will close the duct. Although a murmur may be absent, this is not always the case.

14. BDE
Innocent murmurs are common during childhood, however, a structural cardiac lesion should be excluded unless the following features are clearly present:
- Child free of cardiac symptoms
- Normal single heart sound and a normally split second heart sound (physiological splitting of the second heart sound increases on inspiration especially in the young and fit. Fixed splitting is associated with an ASD and reverse splitting with delayed closure of the aortic valve)
- No added clicks or diastolic murmurs
- Murmur loudest in the supine position and decreased in intensity on assuming and upright posture
- Normal cardiac rhythm and blood pressure

15. ABC
Cannon waves occur when the right atrium contracts against a closed tricuspid valve as may occur consistently in a nodal rhythm or intermittently in atrio-ventricular dissociation. Asymmetrical septal hypertrophy may cause right ventricular outflow obstruction and lead to right atrial hypertrophy with a giant "a" wave, as may pulmonary stenosis.

Practice Exam Answers

16. ABCD
Neonatal presentation of cystic fibrosis may be with meconium ileus, meconium perforation and peritonitis, obstructive jaundice, elevated immunoreactive trypsin or in a positive sweat test in a sibling of a known cystic fibrosis patient. Circulatory collapse may occur in hot weather because of excessive salt losses. Although nasal polyps occur in cystic fibrosis, presentation with them would be unusual as they are usually present after long-standing disease.

17. D
A positive 6 minute exercise test occurs in 80% of children with asthma, and 90–95% if the test is repeated on several occasions. However, exercise-induced asthma usually comes on after 6–10 minutes of exercise. Although the mechanism remains obscure, repeated exercise challenge produces less bronchoconstriction, i.e. there is a refractory period lasting up to one hour. Steroids will only modify the response if given for several weeks prior to exercise, whereas sodium cromoglycate or β_2 stimulants are very effective taken immediately prior to exercise. Histamine has been demonstrated in the blood stream after prolonged exercise.

18. BCDE
Bronchiolitis is an acute infection caused principally by respiratory syncytial virus, other viruses implicated include influenza, parainfluenza and adenovirus. It occurs commonly during the first 6 months of life but is seen throughout the first year. Seasonal epidemics occur with peak incidence in winter and early spring. Commonly the only sign seen on radiographs is a hyperinflated chest. The disease is usually self limiting, but may be more severe in children with underlying cardiac and respiratory problems. Permanent damage after bronchiolitis is rare, but bronchiectasis, bronchiolitis obliterans and McLeod's syndrome are reported after adenoviral pneumonia.

19. BD
Sleep apnoea is an increasing problem. Recognised features include daytime hypersomnolence, intellectual deterioration and morning headache. Apnoeas are longest in REM sleep and are associated with bradycardia. Systemic hypertension and tachycardias occur during arousal.

Practice Exam Answers

20. ABDE
ABO incompatibility is usually much milder than rhesus disease and may occur in the first pregnancy because the mothers "natural" blood group antibodies, although usually IgM, may be IgG antibodies, which can cross the placenta. ABO incompatibility occurs in 20–25% of pregnancies, but haemolytic disease occurs in only 10% of these children. Low antigenicity of the ABO factors in the fetus and new born infant may account for this. The children are often quite normal initially, and Coombs' test may be normal or only weakly positive. Although the jaundice is usually unconjugated, a conjugated hyperbilirubinaemia can occur.

21. AD
Reticulocytosis will be seen in conditions where there is anaemia secondary to red cell destruction, such as rhesus incompatibility or sickle cell disease. In any cause of bone marrow aplasia (Fanconi anaemia=congenital aplastic anaemia) aberrant/depressed bone marrow function is the cause of the anaemia so that reticulocytes, (which are immature precursors of red blood cells) will not be generated and pushed into the circulation.

22. BE
Bleeding time depends mainly on capillary function and platelet numbers and function. It will therefore be normal in haemophilia A and B (Christmas disease). It is characteristically abnormal in von Willebrand's disease. In Henoch-Schönlein purpura, the cutaneous lesions are the result of a small vessel vasculitis.

23. ABE
An important feature of Wilm's tumour is its association with congenital anomalies:
    genitourinary abnormalities   4.4%
    hemihypertrophy   2.9%
    sporadic aniridia   1.1%
It is not associated with familial aniridia or reactions to vaccinations.

24. E
At 12 months a child would be expected to bang bricks together when given them, but not to build a tower of 3 bricks until he or she is 18 months old. Similarly, children would not be expected to feed

Practice Exam Answers

themselves until they are 18 months old, and 10% of 2-year-olds cannot yet do this. Single words are the norm at 12 months, although walking around a cot would be expected from about 10 months onwards. At 15–18 months children start to remove shoes, socks and gloves.

25. ABD
The commonest cause of a large head is a genetic predisposition. This should be verified by measuring parents' head circumference. A large head *per se* is less significant than a head that is deviating upwards on a centile chart, hydrocephalus may be a cause of this. Achondroplastics have large heads from infancy, but other skeletal abnormalities should make this diagnosis obvious. Craniosynostosis will cause a small or abnormally shaped head.

26. CE
In partially treated congenital adrenal hyperplasia, bone age will be advanced. This is often seen in non-salt losing males who are diagnosed relatively late. Similarly, children with Turner's syndrome can get premature closure of their epiphyses, and oestrogen therapy may delay this. Social deprivation has a variety of effects, including delaying physical maturation.

27. D
Eating disorders are a spectrum ranging from anorexia nervosa, through to bulimia nervosa to bulimia and obese binge eating. Anorexia nervosa is characterised by:
- morbid fear of fatness
- a distorted body image
- body weight more than 25% below normal for age
- amenorrhoea in women (often precedes weight loss)

It occurs in both sexes and at all ages. The patients often have a great interest in food, preparing elaborate meals for their families. Laxative, emetic and purgative abuse and excessive exercise are common. Lanugo hair develops.

28. ABCD
Disorganised behaviour is characteristic of the subtype of schizophrenia known as "hebephrenic" schizophrenia in the ICD-10 classification. Delusions of control are a form of "passivity" phenom-

Practice Exam Answers

ena and include "made" feelings, impulses or acts in which the subject feels influenced or controlled by an external force or agency. These are also Schneiderian "First Rank" symptoms of schizophrenia. Mood in schizophrenia may be shallow or inappropriate (incongruous). The ICD-10 description of schizophrenia states that "... intellectual capacity is usually maintained, though certain cognitive deficits may evolve in the course of time ..." Visual hallucinations may occur in schizophrenia but are not characteristic of the disorder.

29. BCD
Autism commonly presents with delayed speech and occurs in 0.7–4.5 per 1000 children. The autistic child is withdrawn, and a history of a delay in social smiling and other social behaviour is often elicited. Eye contact is minimal and the child has compulsive and repetitive routines and play, disruption of which may cause tantrums.

30. ABDE
A wide range of maternal disease can affect the fetus because of
- teratogenic effects of metabolic products of disease (phenylalanine/glucose)
- teratogenic effects of drugs used for treatment (e.g. warfarin)
- antibody transfer (ITP/Graves' disease/myaesthenia).

Conversely, a number of diseases in the mother may be worsened by pregnancy (multiple sclerosis).

31. ABC
Necrotising enterocolitis (NEC) is most common in low birth weight babies, although it occasionally occurs in term infants. It is much less common in infants who have not been fed. The incidence varies widely between centres and the pathophysiology is very poorly understood. Recognised risk factors include: low birth weight, asphyxia, artificial feeds, intrauterine growth retardation, polycythaemia, cardiac and umbilical catheters, early feeding. The aetiology may include: immaturity of bowel transport and motility and decreased host resistance. The importance of infectious agents has never been proved. The colon and ileum are most frequently affected. Approximately 10% of affected infants will develop a stricture and require surgery after NEC. Gut function in the majority of survivors appears normal.

Practice Exam Answers

32. BCDE
Infants with intrauterine growth retardation are predisposed to many perinatal problems. The exception is respiratory distress syndrome, and it is thought that perinatal stress matures their lungs faster. Milder degrees of perinatal asphyxia may cause severe effects because of poor fat and glycogen stores and thus the inability to maintain anaerobic metabolism.

33. ABD
Cryptosporidia characteristically give watery diarrhoea and the disease is rare in children less than 1 year of age. Verotoxin characteristically produces bloody diarrhoea and this may be followed by the haemolytic uraemic syndrome. Diarrhoea associated with *Giardia* and *Campylobacter* may or may not be bloody.

34. AB
In over 90% of otherwise thriving children with recurrent abdominal pain an underlying organic cause is not found. Low residue diets will not help in the majority of cases, although enquiry about diet should be undertaken as parents or the child may have modified the child's diet to try to help the pain and it may not be nutritionally adequate. In the majority, investigations should be limited to urine microscopy and culture and a full blood count and ESR.

35. ABCE
Symptoms of ulcerative colitis begin before the age of 20 in about 15% of patients and although it is described in the neonatal period, it is uncommon pre-adolescence. In most patients the onset is gradual. The impact of the disease is often reflected in the child's general demeanor and the disease itself or its treatment may result in short stature. Extraintestinal signs are less common in adults than children, but about 10% show signs of arthritis, usually of the large joints. Pyoderma gangrenosum, iritis and clubbing are very rare and only seen late in the disease. Anaemia, not polycythaemia occurs.

36. BDE
Eating disorders are a spectrum ranging from anorexia to bulimia. Anorexia can be divided into restrictive and bulimic types. Physical sequelae of anorexia nervosa include hypokalaemia, osteopenia, anaemia, leucopenia and hypothalamo-pituitary-gonadal axis disturbances

with secondary amenorrhoea. Levels of follicle stimulating hormone and luteinising hormone are prepubertal i.e. low. Buccal pigmentation, weight loss and hypokalaemia are features of Addison's disease.

37. BCD
The serum calcium concentration is an important determinant of calcitonin secretion. The main action of calcitonin is to inhibit osteoclastic bone resorption. Calcitonin is a 32 amino acid single chain polypeptide. It is secreted by the C cells of the thyroid (and not the thyroid epithelial cell!). It is these cells which give rise to the malignancy in medullary carcinoma of the thyroid.

38. ABD
Parathyroid hormone (PTH) rises in response to low serum calcium, causing increases in serum calcium and a fall in phosphate. Primary hyperparathyroidism occurs when the excess PTH is inappropriate to the normal plasma calcium level. Secondary or tertiary hyperparathyroidism occurs in chronic renal failure. In pseudohypoparathyroidism there is a receptor defect, so that the raised levels of PTH fail to mobilise calcium. In Paget's disease and multiple myeloma, calcium levels are raised and PTH secretion is suppressed.

39. ACE
The concentration of IgA in colostrum is extremely high, at least 10 times as high as adult serum, but falls rapidly to serum levels after about 4 days of lactation. The IgA of breast milk originates from B cells in breast tissue, which migrate there from gastrointestinal and respiratory mucosal follicles. In addition to protecting the newborn from infection, breast milk antibodies may play a role in establishing the normal gut flora and in preventing allergy, although the mechanism of the latter is unknown. Breast milk also contains a significant number of cells. The majority of these are granulocytes and macrophages, but small numbers of B and T lymphocytes are present.

40. ABCE
The complement proteins are a large family of proteins involved in a wide range of inflammatory reactions. Complement is found in the lesions in extrinsic allergic alveolitis and levels are low in SLE and PSGN, suggesting that complement binding of immune complexes may be important in these diseases. Paroxysmal nocturnal haemo-

Practice Exam Answers

globinuria is due to a defect in lipid-anchored regulatory proteins that include members of the complement family. The aetiology of sarcoidosis is poorly understood but probably involves antigen interaction with T cells and macrophages.

41. CE
There is an increasing body of evidence that MMR vaccination is quite safe in children with egg allergy, although it should be given under supervision where resuscitation facilities are available (See 1996 Immunisation book [green book]). The only neurological contraindication to vaccination is a **progressive** neurological disease. Varicella is a live attenuated vaccine that is only available in the UK on a named basis but is more widely used in the USA and seems to be safe in the immunocompromised. Any mother who is not immune to polio should be vaccinated at the same time as her child and told to take extra care when handling nappies etc. because of the small risk of "vaccine polio" in a non-immune individual.

42. AE
This child has a characteristic history of post streptococcal glomerulonephritis. In nephritis, renal function is impaired such that hypertension and fluid retention occur. The latter may result in pulmonary oedema with the characteristic bat wing shadowing on CXR. Serum C3 levels are usually decreased. There is no specific therapy for this disease, and complete recovery occurs in 95% of children. The normal supportive measures used in acute renal failure should therefore be used. Steroids are the treatment of choice in nephrotic syndrome, in which children are likely to be markedly oedematous with proteinuria and a normal or low blood pressure due to a low intravascular volume.

43. BCD
Renal tubular acidosis may be type I (distal) or type II (proximal). Both types can be primary or secondary and can occur at any time of life. Type II is caused by excess bicarbonate in the urine, and type I by a failure of secretion of hydrogen ions into the urine. In type II urine, pH may fall to low levels in severe systemic acidosis, this does not occur in type I where the urine pH remains above 6 even in severe acidosis. Children often present in early life with polyuria, dehydration, constipation and failure to thrive. Nephrocalcinosis or renal tract calculi occur in 70%.

Practice Exam Answers

44. BE
Minimal change glomerulonephritis has normal light microscopy and immunohistochemical findings. The only abnormalities will be seen on electron microscopy with the fusion of foot processes. Affected children have a highly selective proteinuria of low molecular weight albumin, are normal between relapses and the majority have a normal outcome. 95% of patients initially respond to steroids within 4 weeks, and although 7% continue to relapse into adult life, end stage renal failure "never" occurs.

45. B
Leukaemia and idiopathic scrotal oedema tend to be painless, although considerable swelling and erythema may be present in the latter. Torsion of the testis will give pain and swelling. The appendix of the testis is an embryological remnant of the paramesonephric ducts, it is found at the upper pole of the testis and may become cystic.

46. BCD
Neck rigidity may precede spinal rigidity in polio. Arthritis of the spine occurs in 50% of patients with Still's disease. In cerebellar astrocytoma or medulloblastoma episodes of loss of consciousness with extensor and neck rigidity, pupillary dilation and respiratory abnormalities may occur.

47. BCDE
Newborns have a relatively low glomerular filtration rate and drugs that are excreted renally may accumulate to toxic levels unless given in lower or less frequent doses in the neonate. Aminoglycosides may cause nephro- and ototoxicity *per se* and the addition of other nephrotoxic agents or conditions will exacerbate this tendency. Frusemide is excreted by glomerular filtration and secreted by a weak organic acid tubular mechanism. Its effects may be delayed and prolonged and could therefore precipitate prerenal failure.

48. BCDE
Risk factors for thrombosis include smoking (especially in those over 35 years), hypertension, obesity, diabetes and a family history of heart disease or stroke. Oestrogen free contraceptives have minimal risk of thrombosis. Contraindications to the pill include a history of

Practice Exam Answers

venous or arterial thrombosis, any known pro-thrombotic coagulation abnormality, severe migraine and liver disease.

49. ACD
The earliest complications of diabetes mellitus are seen at around late puberty, with microscopic albuminuria. Isophane is a long-acting insulin. Blood HbA1c or fructosamine reflect the longer term glucose control and are a helpful guide to overall control. Lipohypertrophy may occur if injection sites are not rotated adequately, giving rise to unreliable absorption of insulin, and may be the cause of an apparent escalation of insulin requirements. Lipoatrophy is increasingly rare, it was largely caused by the use of less pure insulins, and its incidence has declined with the introduction of purer animal and recombinant human preparations. Insulin requirements often decrease after diagnosis: the "honeymoon period".

50. ABCD
Children with 21 hydroxylase deficiency may be salt losers, when they have low aldosterone levels, high renin levels and hyponatraemic dehydration, with elevated potassium. ACTH levels will not be high.

51. AD
75% of cases of congenital spherocytosis are autosomal dominant. Vitamin D resistant rickets is one of the few X-linked dominant genes identified. All of the major types of congenital adrenal hyperplasia are autosomal recessive, differences in manifestations between males and females are due to virulisation of females. Hereditary haemorrhagic telangectasia (Osler Weber Rendu) is autosomal dominant, whereas ataxia telangectasia, another inherited disease with telangectasia is inherited in an autosomal recessive fashion. Infantile polycystic kidney disease is inherited in an autosomal recessive manner, the adult form is autosomal dominant, although the adult form may rarely present in infancy.

52. ABD
Fragile X is the commonest cause of mental retardation after Down's syndrome, it affects both males and females and accounts for 10% of all mentally retarded children. The incidence ranges from 03.–1 per 1000 in males and 0.2–0.6 per 1000 in females. Female carriers exhibit a very variable phenotype, from normality to symptoms very

Practice Exam Answers

similar to classical male fragile X. The defect lies within the FMR-1 gene on the long arm of the X chromosome. The number of CGG repeats adjacent to the promoter region in the normal gene is stable and is up to 50. In fragile X the number of repeats increases in a stepwise fashion resulting in ultimate loss of expression.

53. BE
The majority of defects with teratogens occur in the first trimester, at the time of maximal organogenesis, 5–8 weeks. Problems within the first couple of weeks are likely to cause failure of implantation or early miscarriage. In both sexes the mesonephric (Wolffian) duct gives rise to the ureteric bud (forming the ureter, calyces and collecting tubules). In the male it also becomes the duct of the epididymis, the vas deferens and the seminal vesicle, whilst this portion of the mesonephric duct largely disappears in the female. The uterus and vagina are formed from the paramesonephric ducts, which largely degenerate in the male. The thyroid develops from the floor of the primitive pharynx and migrates down towards the larynx. Neural crest cells give rise to a range of cells including: cells of the posterior root ganglion, sensory ganglia of cranial nerves, autonomic ganglia, Schwann cells, cells of the suprarenal medulla and melanocytes.

54. AD
Malnutrition is divided into marasmus, with normal serum albumin, and Kwashiokor (protein energy malnutrition) with characteristically low albumin. The latter contributes to the oedema seen in these children, oedema of internal organs may occur before other oedema and oedema may mask the degree of weight loss seen in these children. Blood glucose levels may be low, but glucose tolerance is often "diabetic" in type. Potassium, magnesium and vitamin A deficiencies are common. Immune responses and thyroid and other hormones (e.g. growth hormones) are deficient.

55. A
Any child with a permanent squint should be referred for ophthalmological assessment because of the risk of amblyopia developing. A cover test detects a squint. Similarly, visual acuity should be corrected with glasses as early as possible to assist the normal development of the child.

Practice Exam Answers

56. ABD
Most patients with SLE have antibodies to double-stranded DNA, although their absence does not exclude the diagnosis. Deposition of complement and immunoglobulin is usually found on the glomerular basement in SLE nephritis, with haematoxylin bodies being found in areas of inflammation. Lymphopenia may be seen, which results in a relative, but not an absolute neutrophilia.

57. BD
For a normal distribution: mean = median = mode. Observations are distributed symmetrically about the mean value (i.e the data scatter identically on both sides of the mean). 95% of observations lie within two standard deviations of the mean (so, by definition, only 5% of observations lie beyond two standard deviations from the mean).

58. BDE
Umbilical hernias are most frequently seen in low birth weight and black infants. Although it is a feature of hypothyroidism, most infants with umbilical hernias do not have hypothyroidism. The majority of hernias will disappear by one year of age, strangulation is rare, and operation is only indicated if the hernia persists until age 3–4, causes symptoms or becomes progressively larger.

59. ADE
Serous otitis media may recur throughout childhood, especially in the winter months, and cause impairment of hearing and subsequent learning difficulties. It usually causes symptoms in the child, but may resolve spontaneously in a proportion of children. Breast feeding has been shown to be protective, as is having non-smoking parents.

60. ABCE
Atrial natriuretic peptide, initially isolated from the atrium of the heart has numerous effects. The major effects are stimulation of natriuresis and diuresis by the kidney through its haemodynamic and tubular effects. In addition, ANP causes vasodilatation and fluid volume reduction by direct actions on vascular smooth muscle cells, and inhibition of secretion of hormones, such as aldosterone, from adrenal cortex and noradrenaline from peripheral adrenergic neurons. Centrally mediated effects (there are ANP receptors in the brain) on the regulation of fluid volume may also be important.

PASTEST BOOKS FOR MRCP 1 PAEDIATRICS

MRCP Part 1 Paediatric MCQ Revision Book
Ian Maconochie MRCP, Jo Wilmshurst MRCP ISBN 0 906896 39 8
This MCQ Revision book contains:
- 300 MCQs arranged by subject which are based on the new MRCP Part 1 Paediatric syllabus
- answers and extended teaching explanations
- comprehensive revision index
- one complete Practice Examination of 60 MCQs

This combination of subject-based MCQs and a complete practice paper will make this book invaluable to all candidates.

MRCP Part 1 Paediatric MCQ Practice Exams
Ian Maconochie MRCP ISBN 0 906896 59 2
This new Paediatric book contains:
- six complete MCQ Practice Papers (360 MCQs)
- an authentic combination of paediatric, general medicine and basic science questions
- answers and detailed teaching notes for every question
- comprehensive index plus MCQ subject listings

An invaluable and eagerly awaited book for the paediatric exam.

Explanations to the Royal College Red Booklet
ISBN 0 906896 54 1 *available by mail order only*
Answers and expert teaching notes related to the RCP red book of sample paediatric exam questions
Indispensable insight and guidance for all MRCP Part 1 Paediatric candidates.

For full details of the range of PasTest books and courses available for MRCP Part 1 candidates, contact PasTest today:

PasTest, Egerton Court, Parkgate Estate,
Knutsford, Cheshire WA16 8DX

Telephone: 01565 755226 Fax: 01565 650264
e-mail: pastest@dial.pipex.com
Web site: http://ds.dial.pipex.com/pastest

PASTEST COURSES FOR MRCP 1 PAEDIATRICS

PasTest are the leading independent specialists in postgraduate medical education. Over the past 25 years, we have helped many thousands of doctors to pass postgraduate medical examinations. Our popular six-day MRCP Part 1 Paediatric courses are run three times a year at convenient venues in London and Manchester. PasTest MRCP Part 1 courses are very popular and have a high reputation. This is quite simply because the majority of Doctors who attend our courses then go on to pass their exams.

PasTest Part 1 Paediatric courses are:

- ✓ intensive, practical and exam oriented
- ✓ designed to strengthen exam technique
- ✓ interactive and entertaining
- ✓ the key to exam success

When you attend our course, each delegate receives course notes consisting of approximately 250 pages of exam-based MCQs with answers and comprehensive notes, plus many explanatory handouts.

PasTest Paediatric courses identify the key areas for revision by:

- ✓ working through past Membership questions
- ✓ updating your knowledge of basic sciences
- ✓ comparing your standard to others on the course
- ✓ enabling you to work out your own profile of strengths and weaknesses

For full details of forthcoming dates and venues, please contact

PasTest, Egerton Court, Parkgate Estate,
Knutsford, Cheshire WA16 8DX

Telephone: 01565 755226 Fax: 01565 650264
e-mail: pastest@dial.pipex.com
Web site: http://ds.dial.pipex.com/pastest